Alternative Health Care for Women

This book is both a self-help guide and a survey of therapies particularly suitable for women. It includes advice and information about preventive health care, women's illnesses, fertility and reproduction, and choosing the best treatment for you.

Alternative Health Care for Women

A woman's guide to self-help
treatments and alternative
therapies
by
Patsy Westcott

THORSONS PUBLISHING GROUP
Wellingborough, Northamptonshire

Rochester, Vermont

First published 1987

© PATSY WESTCOTT 1987

British Library Cataloguing in Publication Data

Westcott, Patsy
  Alternative health care for women: a
  woman's guide to self-help treatments and
  alternative therapies.
  1. Women — Diseases — Treatment
  I. Title
  615.5   RG126

  ISBN 0-7225-1360-7

Reproduced, printed and bound in Great Britain by
Hazell Watson & Viney Limited,
Member of the BPCC Group,
Aylesbury, Bucks

10 9 8 7 6 5 4 3 2 1

Contents

Acknowledgements

My thanks go first of all to the many alternative and orthodox practitioners who gave freely of their time and expertise. Next, and no less important, I thank all those friends who shared their own personal experiences and views, and endured endless kitchen table discussions, which helped enormously in clarifying my own ideas.

My thanks, too, to the staff at the Women's Health Information Centre for allowing me the use of their collection; and to Pilgrim Hospital Medical Library, especially Shirley Brewster, for making available books and articles, and putting up with a chronic late returner.

I write as a woman first and foremost and a journalist next. Since the book is intended for a general readership, technical vocabulary and jargon have been kept to a minimum. Wherever possible I have used popular names for illnesses, rather than the medical term. Academic references have been judiciously pruned, too, to make for easier reading.

Suggestions for further reading, and sources of help and information have been included in the text as they arise. I hope this makes for easy reference.

The book is intended as a taster. If it gives you a flavour of what alternative therapy is about, and whets your appetite for more, I will have succeeded in what I set out to do. If you have any personal experience of any of the therapies mentioned or ideas arising from the book, do let me know. Any faults or omissions are, of course my own.

I'd like to thank Fay Franklin of Thorsons, for her patience and support as an editor. And last, but by no means least, I am grateful to my two daughters Lucy and Kate for keeping me going with cups of tea, for putting up with yet another ready meal, and for continuing to love a mother whose mind must have sometimes seemed to be more on homoeopathy than the school concert. This book is for them.

PATSY WESTCOTT

Women and the health services

Women are no strangers to the doctor's surgery. During our reproductive years we visit the doctor twice as often as men. We suffer more illness than men. And we gobble more pills, both of the on-prescription and over-the-counter variety, than men. Many of these are for mood-altering drugs such as anti-depressants and tranquillizers. According to one survey a staggering 33 per cent of women between the ages of 45 and 49 are on such medication, compared with just 10 per cent of men. In fact, in the 1980s, women are both the main consumers and main providers of health care. Why?

Part of the reason we seem to spend so much time in our doctor's company is that so many of our basic biological functions such as menstruation, pregnancy and childbirth, the menopause, seem to come under the umbrella of medicine. We have to visit our doctor if we don't want a baby. We have to see him again (I say 'he' advisedly since most doctors are still men) if we do want a baby. And once we become mothers, as guardians of our family's welfare, we spend many hours in clinics waiting for check-ups, immunizations and dealing with everyday ailments.

What's more — despite improvements in living standards, improved housing, better diet, more effective birth control, and safer childbirth which have meant that today's woman can expect to live twice as long as her great-great grandmother — the circumstances of women's lives still lead to a lot of chronic illness. In particular, women are prey to depressive illness. And, as any doctor will tell you, this takes up a fair share of their time. I'll be looking at this whole question in more detail in the section dealing with mental health (page 94).

Yet, despite the fact that many of us seem to spend so much of our lives lurking around doctors' waiting rooms, there's a strong feeling on the part of many women that they get a raw deal from the medical profession. Several surveys have highlighted the discontent many of us feel with our doctors. Lack of time, not listening to what you have to say, and not giving sufficient information, are some typical complaints. Here are just a few of the comments taken from a selection of these surveys:

'Every time I come away from my G.P. it's with a prescription and feeling frustrated and dissatisfied.'

'I was telling him about my irritation and he kept looking at his watch. He didn't know what was wrong with me but said, "Since I haven't got much time, I'll treat you for thrush for the moment".'

'I would have liked to have known more about why my body was behaving the way it was.'

'In hospital they put that plastic wrist band on, and you become a slab of meat.'

Another survey, this time conducted by a medical sociologist, suggests that many of us have difficulty talking to our doctors. Fifty five per cent of the women, and forty-two per cent of the men studied, became speechless once they entered the hallowed grounds of the doctor's surgery. And this was worse if they were 'feeling nervous'. Those who got the most out of their doctors had both knowledge and confidence, the report concludes.

The fact is that the health care we get is in the main delivered by doctors who by virtue of their sex, background and training are often ill-equipped to deal with many of the problems we take to them. Women's bodies, as portrayed in many of the textbooks doctors use, are little more than a pair of ovaries with a human being attached.

One criticism sometimes levelled at orthodox medicine by those favouring alternative therapies is that it sees the body simply as a collection of parts and doesn't take into account dimensions which aren't purely physical. This isn't strictly true. In fact, doctors *do* use other criteria when dealing with patients' problems, but these are rarely brought into the light of day. Let's imagine that you visit your doctor complaining of migraine, for example. The advice you get will depend not purely on your physical symptoms, but on a whole host of unacknowledged factors such as the way you look, dress and speak, as well as your doctor's ideas about the respective roles of men and women. This is brought out in an entertaining, but also somewhat alarming account of her 'career' as a migraine patient by Sally MacIntyre. Her first doctor saw her migraine as a physical complaint. She was sent off with a drug and advice on anticipating and dealing with attacks. Her next doctor interpreted it as a conflict between career and home — no prizes for guessing which he advised her to give up. Even more unlucky was her encounter with a doctor who saw the migraine as the result of deep-seated personality difficulties:

My migraine resulted from my not having a boyfriend, sublimating my desire for children in postgraduate studies and having over-strong internalized guilt and achievement strivings. When I became depressed lest these were true, the migraine was ascribed to depressive tendencies!

This isn't to suggest that any or all these explanations might not contain a grain of truth, but as Helen Roberts remarks in her book *The Patient Patient* (Pandora): '. . . going to the doctor's may not just be a matter of getting a prescription, but also of getting a prescription for the appropriate way to lead your life.'

The difficulties women encounter with their doctors partly explain why so many are looking to alternative therapies, but these aren't the only reasons. One of the biggest nails in the coffin for orthodox medicine has been the increase in side-effects caused by many modern drugs: the 'iatrogenic' or doctor-induced diseases.

Women in particular have been the victims of some of the more dramatic failures of modern pharmacology. Thalidomide, responsible for the birth of many thousands of handicapped children, was a drug given to pregnant women. Less well-known perhaps is DES (diethylstilboestrol) a synthetic hormone administered to large numbers of expectant mothers who had suffered previous miscarriages. This resulted in the development of vaginal and genital cancers in their children. More recently still, Debendox, a drug which used to be prescribed to treat morning sickness, has been withdrawn on suspicion of causing birth defects.

Just as worrying is the evidence that despite the best that modern medicine has to offer, we're far from cracking some of the most common complaints that afflict women. Survival rates for breast cancer have barely inched up in the last 50 years, despite ever-more sophisticated treatments. And while thousands of pounds are poured into high-profile illnesses such as heart-disease, the everyday but debilitating problems such as thrush, cystitis, menstrual problems, and the vague but troublesome aches and pains that affect so many of us are still far from being adequately treated.

However, despite all this it's not all gloom and doom. The realization that modern medicine doesn't have all the answers has caused patients and doctors alike to explore alternatives to conventional treatment. Therapies such as homoeopathy, acupuncture, osteopathy, chiropractic and a host of others once dismissed to the lunatic fringe have come in from the cold. And despite the unfavourable report on the alternative therapies published in 1986 by the British Medical Association, both public and professional interest in these therapies is strong.

In fact a survey of G.Ps carried out for *The Times* newspaper group in 1985 found that a high proportion actually practised some type of alternative therapy, a further 26 per cent had received alternative treatment themselves, while 57 per cent were interested in learning to practise some form of alternative treatment. The British Holistic Medical Association, an organization formed in 1983, for doctors and other healthcare workers, aims to bring together both orthodox and alternative therapies, while the Research Council for Complementary Medicines is subsidizing a number of research projects designed to test the effectiveness of various therapies.

Another promising development is self-help health care. Spurred on in part by the women's movement, women have been getting together to find out how their bodies work and to take some of the mystique out of medical care. Part of this exploration has been to investigate what the various alternatives have to offer.

So what is alternative health care? What can it do for you? Alternative health care can't work miracles, and you should be extremely suspicious of any practitioner who claims it can. However, it can be an effective first-line of treatment for a number of common complaints. It can also be a useful second string if you are undergoing conventional treatment.

Alternative health care can help you stay healthy, treat some illnesses, and relieve many conditions for which there is no cure. Basic to the alternative health care approach are several ideas:

● The body is finely balanced and illness is caused by it getting out of balance.

● If you become ill the body has the capacity to heal itself, given the right support and encouragement.

● Disease is often a result of the way we live our lives.

But alternative health care isn't just about choosing an unconventional therapy. It's about looking at health and illness in a new way. And it's about examining the part our life styles play in the breakdown of health.

In the rest of this book I explain how alternative health care can work for you. The first part looks at how you can care for yourself so as to stay as healthy as possible. Part 2 goes into the common illnesses that affect women, and the options for treatment both orthodox and alternative. Part 3 looks at fertility and reproduction, and how alternative therapies can help you conceive, take care of yourself in pregnancy and give birth. There's a section too on the menopause. In Part 4 you'll find a rundown of the various alternative therapies and what illnesses they are especially useful in treating. There are tips on what to look for in an alternative practitioner and how to avoid cowboys.

Useful books on women's health:

Our Bodies, Ourselves: A Health Book by and for Women, Angela Phillips and Jill Rakusen, (Penguin).
The New Guide to Women's Health, Dr Norma Williams, and Hetty Einzig, (Macdonald).

Both fairly orthodox — for information on alternative therapy for women, see end of Introduction to Part 4.

PART ONE

Staying Healthy

A Sense of Well-Being

Not only are women the main consumers of health services, they're also the main providers of health care. Whether as nurses, social workers, ancillary workers of all kinds, or as wives, mothers and daughters, we spend a good deal of time caring for others. But all too often, we neglect our own health. We work long hours both outside and inside the home, we rush around trying to fit everything in . . . and then, we smoke, drink or go on eating binges to cope with all the pressures.

Many alternative therapies are based on the idea that health is damaged by ignoring, repressing or denying our basic needs. Sometimes it's only when we experience an unexpected miscarriage, a relationship going wrong, an episode of chronic illness or even the development of cancer that we stop short and take a look at our own lives.

That's not to say that it's your fault if you fall ill, nor that you should be in tip-top health the whole time. There's nothing 'bad' about being ill. Women blame themselves about enough things, without beating themselves around the head for falling sick. In fact a spell of illness or a bout of depression may often be the one thing that forces us to take a much-needed break. Being ill can give you a breathing space, a time to take stock of who you are and where you are going.

But that said, most of us would prefer to be well. And though alternative health care can't solve the problems of insufficient money, pollution, where you live, the work you do, and many of the other causes of ill health, it can help you to take care of yourself, so that you are better able to withstand disease. You don't have to wait for your health to break down to make changes in your life. You can start now to tune in to your own physical, social and spiritual needs. Alternative health care means paying attention to what you eat, getting enough exercise, feeding your mind and feeling a sense of fulfilment in life.

In a world where women in particular suffer from a lack of choice and power, looking after our own health and knowing when to seek help can give us a valuable sense of control. It can also give you extra energy and confidence to get involved in practical things that might change life for the better if you wish, for both yourself and others.

The idea most of us have about health is that it is an absence of illness. But how many of us who aren't exactly ill can say that we feel really healthy either? *The General Household Survey* of 1979 revealed that seven out of ten women had some health problem at the time of the interview. A survey carried out in a women's magazine in the same year opened a whole Pandora's box of aches and pains, headache, depression, palpitations, indigestion, rheumatism, chronic tiredness, high blood-pressure and sore throats, to mention just a few. There's no evidence to suggest things are any better today. The fact is many of us feel slightly under par for much of the time. And while illness is part of the normal flux of life, many of us experience an ebbing vitality and a lack of 'zest'. A sense of well-being can be yours whatever your age or disabilities. It comes from knowing who you are and where you are going.

Making changes

Change calls for action. So how do you start? The first step is to take a hard look at your life. The key to health from this perspective lies in giving due weight to all the different aspects of your life. That means not just taking care of your body by attending to what you eat, taking enough exercise and so on, but also looking at your social relationships, your mental life and your spiritual needs. This last need is quite difficult for most of us to understand. Traditionally such needs have gone under the banner of religion. With the decline in church-going and organized religion, spiritual dimensions of life have tended to be ignored or dismissed as irrelevant. But whether you subscribe to an accepted faith or not, the truth is we all need to make sense of our lives and to feel a sense of direction and purpose.

Ready . . .

Start off by imagining how you would like your life to be if you had completely free choice. This is your first taste of an alternative technique called visualization, or guided meditation. Don't censor yourself at this point. If you've always had a fantasy of going off and living on a Greek island with a couple of goats for company, go ahead and indulge it. You'll be able to work out what's realistic and what isn't later. But you can't decide how to achieve what you really want until you know what it is.

. . . Get set . . .

Once you've thought about how you would like your life to be, you can start to inject a spot of realism into your programme. It may help at this point to write it all down. Set yourself goals. Say what you would like to be doing in five years' time, one year, six months and three months. This will help you plan, and more importantly, it will help put time under your control. Not having enough time to do what we want to do is one of the major causes of stress — and of ill health.

Be specific and try to get a balance between the various different areas of your life. For instance don't just say 'I want to get more exercise', say 'I'm going to go swimming every Tuesday evening between 7 and 8 p.m.'

. . . Go!

Once you've got your plan you can start to put it into practice. You're more likely to succeed if you bear the following tips in mind:

● Be realistic. It might not be possible to take a job at the moment if that is your ambition, because you can't find a childminder, haven't the right training or whatever. But you could perhaps take a further education course, look at childcare options in your area, get together with someone else to swap childcare. In the meantime, is there anything else that would satisfy that need — for instance, getting involved in a community group?

● Be practical. Unless you're very self-disciplined you're not going to trek across town on a winter evening to that yoga class. Is there anything nearer home you could do?

Body: What is right for you in the way of diet and exercise? See the chapters on these for some ideas. Are there any health problems that need sorting out? What alternative therapies might be able to help you? See Parts 2 and 4 for hints on these. Beware of becoming what holistic doctor Laurence LeShan calls a 'holistic athlete', jumping from one therapy to another in the hope it will solve all your problems. Remember true change can only come from within you.

Mind: Many of us take it for granted that our mental powers will automatically deteriorate as we get old. Yet research shows that using the brain cells actually stops them degenerating. Even those of us who are in good physical shape may neglect our mental well-being. Don't. For others the approach to physical health can be made via the mind. For ideas on this see the section on mind-body therapies.

Relationships: Research shows that women are more at risk of depression if they don't have a close confiding relationship. Improving the quality of your relationships may mean sorting out with a partner what you really want from your partnership, and reassessing other relationships that have become stale and dead. It can mean recognizing the ways in which you yourself contribute to rigid patterns. It may even mean breaking out of a relationship that has become dull and stultifying, or deciding to make changes in it.

Deciding to seek psychotherapy, joining a co-counselling group, or exploring other alternative therapies can help you be clear about some of these points. The Women's Therapy Centre, 6 Manor Gardens, London N7, run courses and weekend workshops on a number of topics such as 'Leaving a Relationship', 'Sisters', 'Depression', to help women in the process of coming to grips with their lives.

Spirit: Specific techniques such as yoga, t'ai chi, meditation or creative activities such as dance, drama, music, art, writing, even prayer can help create a sense of greater awareness and meaning in life.

Although I've divided all these areas up for the sake of convenience, they don't exist in isolation. Your aim is to achieve a balance in all areas of your life. The next sections will help you do this.

● Know yourself. Take into account your own strengths and weaknesses. Are you the sort who will stick religiously to a jogging routine, or would you be better off trying to do some other sort of exercise say two or three times a week? For further ideas on this see the chapter on exercise.

● Take it a step at a time. Even positive changes like going on holiday are stressful. Don't let getting healthy become another stick with which to beat yourself.

● Be prepared for setbacks. You're bound not to meet your goals from time to time, so be kind to yourself. If you constantly fail

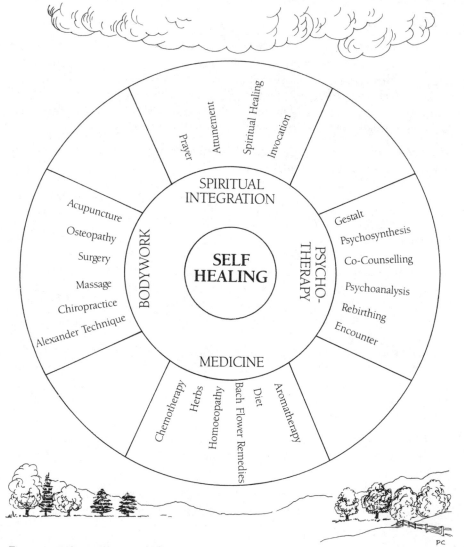

Figure 1: Holistic Health Wheel.

to reach a target it's not because you're no good. Perhaps you're being too ambitious. Could you do something different, or break down what you've set yourself to do into smaller, simpler steps?

● Get others in your life on your side. If you've decided to set aside twenty minutes a day for meditating, arrange for your partner, a friend or neighbour to look after the children, organize a game for them and make sure they understand that you are not to be interrupted.

●Beware of becoming a fanatic. A little bit of what you fancy can only do you good.

● Live in the present. Begin by making small changes that you can easily make straightaway. And don't wait to start living until you've got a better job, stopped smoking, taken up exercise or whatever.

● Learn to listen to yourself. Be aware of your own feelings. Your dreams, intuitions, tastes and preferences, what you like and dislike are all important messages about you. With practice you can use them to guide you into making the right choices for you.

Barriers to change

It isn't always easy to change. Habits and patterns of behaviour build up gradually over long periods of time. Other people's expectations of how women should live their lives often lie at the root of our problems. The fashionable ideal of the perfect figure forces us to starve ourselves and contort our shape. Images of the perfect wife and mother isolate many women in the home. Fear that we're the only ones to shout at our children, stick them in front of the television or feed them junk food cuts us off further from others in the same situation.

Making changes involves a degree of risk too. And many of us have a lot invested in staying the way we are. It only takes a child to say 'I don't like it now you go to evening class' to make most of us crumple. Keeping a sense of balance helps and not trying to do too much at once. So does meeting and talking with other women. Find out if there's a women's health group, or other women's group near you. I'll be looking some more at some of these barriers to change and how you can overcome them in the rest of the book.

Back to basics

You are what you eat

The food we eat is one of the cornerstones of alternative health care. The role of diet in chronic and degenerative disease, allergies, behaviour problems and a whole host of other nasties has been exhaustively chronicled. What's perhaps less well publicized is why so many of us find it hard to follow all the good advice.

Women are the great providers. We're the ones who, on the whole, buy, prepare and cook most of the family's food. But despite all this it's one of the areas where many of us feel particularly out of control. And feeling out of control is one of the major sources of stress, which in turn, is believed by many alternative practitioners to be the root of most illness.

On the one hand we're bombarded with advice on what we should eat. On the other, millions of pounds are poured into persuading us to buy products, many of which are patently unhealthy. At the same time we have to juggle the competing demands of different family members and make it all fit the budget.

A report from York University showed that for many families a 'proper meal' is still meat and two veg, with sweets and puddings a reward for eating up. And, despite women's liberation, many of us are still caught up in the idea that the way to a man's heart is through his stomach. Add on the fact that the kids won't eat anything unless it's fried or smothered in ketchup, and that you are on a diet, and it's small wonder that family meal times are the traditional time for punch-ups!

For many women their role as provider and consumer of food is tied up with feelings of who they are. The women in the York study saw it as their job to prepare the meals and wash-up. What's more, if you're at home all day, preparing and serving up dinner may be one of your few creative outlets. If the family turn up their noses at what you've spent hours lovingly slaving over a hot stove making, it's hardly surprising if you feel a failure. Food then is often a measure of our 'success' as wives and mothers. And if you're slimming, resisting tempting goodies becomes a measure of your 'success' as a woman. So you can see there's far more to food than eating a good diet.

So what's wrong with the food we eat nowadays? And what can you do about it? Although there seems to be more choice than ever before, often it is between one variety of junk food and another. You've only to examine the shelves of the local supermarket to see just how much of what we eat is processed in some way. Buying whole foods and additive-free products usually means paying more. And even those

that are labelled 'additive-free' may have hidden preservatives — in the flour say of an 'additive-free' pizza. The good news is that some shops are bowing to consumer pressure and stocking organically grown vegetables and free-range eggs, albeit at somewhat inflated prices. One way around this is to buy in bulk, or to see whether there are any food co-ops in your area.

To supplement or not to supplement?

The fact that we all eat too much fat, refined sugar and starches, and too little fibre and fresh fruit and vegetables can hardly have escaped anyone's notice in the last few years.

In the last 50 years or so, a complex food industry has grown up, making available a whole range of foods that take up less shelf-space, keep longer and take less time to cook. The problem is that processing destroys many essential nutrients. Many alternative practitioners and nutritionally oriented therapists argue that, because of this and modern methods of factory farming, even those of us who are apparently well-fed could be short of essential vitamins and minerals. Even fresh foods, they say, are low in nutritional value. They may be contaminated with lead from the atmosphere or aluminium from cooking utensils. All of which can lead to deficiencies and excesses of vitamins and minerals that cause all manner of diseases (for more about this see specific illnesses in Part 2). The answer, according to these experts, is vitamin and mineral supplements.

The whole question of supplementation marks the great divide between orthodox doctors and many alternative practitioners. Conventional dieticians and nutritionists, and many naturopaths, claim that so long as you getting a balanced diet there's no need for supplements. Supplements, too, are big business as you can see if you wander down the aisle of your local health food shop.

But the supplementation story is far from clear-cut. A lack of vitamins and minerals may well cause deficiency diseases, but an excess can actually be harmful. The efficacy of megadoses of vitamin C, for example, once hailed as the great cure-all for everything from the common cold to cancer, has been challenged. What's more, too much vitamin C may lead to kidney stones in susceptible people, and can cause withdrawal effects if used for more than one or two weeks. (If you are taking large doses, wean yourself off gradually.) And megadoses of vitamin C in early pregnancy have been found to put women at greater risk of miscarriage.

Methods of testing for vitamin and mineral deficiency or excess are fraught with all sorts of difficulties, not least because no one seems to be able to decide what the recommended daily allowances should be. And in many cases we don't know whether a disease or condition causes deficiency or whether it's the other way round.

Finally, nutrients don't work in isolation. Vitamin C, for instance is needed for iron absorption. Zinc and magnesium work together Adding extra vitamins or minerals willy-nilly can throw the body out of balance. Any supplement you take needs to be carefully tailored to you as an individual.

It's all very confusing isn't it? So should you supplement or not? The list below shows times when you might be short of certain nutrients. If you think you need a supplement consult a practitioner with a special interest in nutrition.

Do I need a supplement?

If you think you may need a supplement the following rule of thumb guide can help you decide. Women who may need extra vitamins or minerals are:

☐ Those who eat an unbalanced diet — for instance if you're a strict vegan, hate raw vegetables, or are excluding certain foods from your diet because of allergy.

☐ Those who are slimming especially if overall intake is below 1,200 calories a day. If you're dieting you may well be low in vitamins A, C, B_6, calcium, iron, magnesium.

☐ Those who have heavy periods. You may need extra calcium because of the risk of osteoporosis (see menopause chapter). This should be taken with magnesium to make calcium intake more effective. You may also be in need of extra iron.

☐ Those who smoke or drink heavily. In this case you will probably need extra vitamin C, vitamins B_6 and B_{12}, thiamin, riboflavin, folic acid, magnesium and zinc.

☐ Those who are pregnant and breast-feeding. For further details see the chapter on pregnancy.

☐ Those who are over 60, especially if you are eating a restricted diet because of lack of money, or disability or ill-health.

☐ Those who have to take regular medication for a chronic ailment; e.g., cortisone can rob the body of calcium. If you regularly take over-the counter medicines (aspirin for instance increases the body's need for folic acid, vitamin C, iron). The Pill can cause a shortage of B_6.

☐ If you've recently been ill or are convalescent. Certain illnesses and infections can rob the body of nutrients.

Rules for taking supplements

● Don't take isolated vitamins or minerals without the advice of a qualified practitioner.

● Always take the supplement with your meals.

● If you buy a multi-vitamin/multi-mineral supplement go for one with a wide and balanced variety of nutrients.

● Don't expect vitamins and minerals to make up for poor eating habits.

● If in doubt consult a qualified practitioner.

Healthy diet guidelines

So what should you eat? And how do you ensure that you are getting a healthy diet? The following guidelines will help you find your way through the diet maze. I've also included a list of minerals and vitamins, so you can see what they are and what they do. If you aim to choose as varied a diet as you can you shouldn't go far wrong.

● Step up your intake of wholegrain cereals, brown rice, wholemeal bread, wholemeal or buckwheat pasta.

● Eat plenty of fresh fruit and vegetables.

● Eat more raw food — some experts claim that 60 per cent of our diet should be raw.

● Avoid storing food for too long. Fruit and vegetables lose nutrients very quickly and

other foods can develop harmful organisms the longer they are stored.

● Cut down on animal fats found in red meat, hard cheeses and so on.

● Go for white meats such as chicken and game animals e.g. rabbit.

● Buy oils high in polyunsaturates such as sunflower. Cook in oil rather than fat.

● Cut out fried foods. Grill, steam, or stew instead.

● Avoid sugary foods, biscuits, cakes, sweets.

● Eat more fish. Fish is low in fat, and fish oils seem to protect against heart disease. Recent evidence suggests that a diet high in fish oils may help prevent premature births.

● Eat more vegetable proteins such as beans, chickpeas, nuts, seeds. Incidentally, the protein value of pulses is increased by combining them with a grain product e.g. dahl and brown rice.

● Don't re-use cooking oils.

● Cut processed foods of all kinds to the very minimum.

● Drink less coffee, tea, cocoa, fizzy drinks. The caffeine in these can make you edgy as well as preventing the body from absorbing certain nutrients (vitamin B_1, thiamin). It's also, according to some practitioners, a factor in hypoglycaemia (low blood sugar) which is responsible for making us feel low.

● Drink more herb teas, fruit juices, bottled water.

Changing to a healthier diet will be easier if you go slowly. Try out new foods when you are feeling relaxed. If you lead a busy life — and who doesn't — invest in a pressure cooker. This takes a lot of the time out of cooking pulses. If you can afford it a freezer is also invaluable. Finally, remember, *how* you eat is almost as important as what you eat. Go to your meals in a relaxed frame of mind.

Additives

Food can be something of a problem if you're in the food industry. It's not uniform in shape, size or colour; it doesn't look tempting unless it's morning fresh; it goes off; and when it's gone off it smells! So what do you do? You process it. The trouble is, processing destroys many essential nutrients which you then have to replace by using synthetic ones, along with dyes, flavourings and preservatives, designed to make the food taste 'better' and look more palatable.

There are at least 3,500 additives in the food we eat in this country. Of these only 400 have been properly tested and have legal controls over their use. Many of them have been banned in other countries for health reasons. And some 40 of the food additives our manufacturers use have come under direct suspicion of causing cancer. Cancer experts Richard Doll and Richard Peto in *The Causes of Cancer* (Oxford University Press), claim that as many as 13,000 cancer deaths in this country each year are caused by food additives.

As women, the additives problem affects us particularly. Women working in the food processing industry in Finland were shown in one study to have a higher risk of miscarriage. And additives have been blamed too for birth defects, still births and lowered fertility. We still don't know how today's plethora of additives might affect future generations.

What's more the foods liked by kids —

crisps, jelly, ice cream, squashes and fizzy drinks — are some of those highest in additives. Children may be especially at risk from their harmful effects. Their immature immune systems mean they are less able to cope with poisons, which, in their smaller bodies, may have a greater effect. Eczema, asthma, diabetes, hyperactivity, diarrhoea, stomach pains, fits, rhinitis, mouth ulcers, vaginal discharge and aches and pains, are just some of the complaints laid at the door of additives by some researchers.

Apart from these specific problems, additives can affect your body's ability to absorb nutrients from food. Additives E220-227, for instance, can destroy vitamin B_1, essential for a healthy nervous system. Other additives bind to nutrients such as iron and calcium so our bodies are unable to use them. Small wonder so many complaints can be tracked back to the food we eat. And all this can be seen as further evidence of the lack of control we have over our lives.

So what can you do if you are worried? On an individual level eat as much fresh and unprocessed food as you can, and label-watch. There are now several books on the market (see below). You can badger your supermarket and food manufacturers to provide additive-free foods; bring the matter to the attention of any groups you belong to, and write to your M.P. At present there are two new big research projects going on into the effects of additives on our health. In the meantime — watch that label!

Further information:
Fact (Food Additives Campaign Team) Room W, 25 Horsell Road, London N5 1XL. London Food Commission, PO Box 291, London N5 1DU.
E for Additives, Maurice Hanssen, (Thorsons).

Irradiation — a new peril?

The furore over additives has caused manufacturers to look to new ways of preserving food. In Holland and elsewhere high intensities of X-rays are used to prevent fresh food from deteriorating. At present this is banned here, but there are signs that the ban may be lifted.

Irradiation destroys the nutritional value of foods. A sub-committee of The Advisory Committee on Irradiated and Novel Foods (how is that for a mouthful?) set up by the DHSS to investigate the whole matter, discovered losses of vitamin B_1 (thiamin), folic acid, vitamins C, K and E. What's more, irradiation can affect the composition and taste of food, so that further additives are necessary.

Even more worrying is the suggestion that food may be at greater rather than less risk of being contaminated because of irradiation. This is because the process can mask signs that food is going off. It also produces chemical subtances, called radiolytic products, that aren't naturally present in foods. We don't really know what the effects of these are.

What foods will be affected? The main ones will be cereals, spices, fruit, vegetables, chicken, shellfish and other meat.

Further information:
Food Irradiation: The Facts by Tony Webb and Dr Tim Lang (Thorsons).

Going vegetarian

Vegetarians usually enjoy excellent health. Vegetarian women are less at risk of breast cancer. And cancer of all kinds seems to be less common in people who don't eat meat. There's also evidence that a vegetarian diet can help sort out menstrual problems, especially if it contains a large number of raw foods.

A recent study by an Australian team of naturopaths looked into the nutritional status of the 'new vegetarians' people who had chosen to go vegetarian for health reasons. They looked at lifestyle, nutrition and level of illness, and carried out blood and biochemical tests. The 'new vegetarians' were well up in vitamin C, B_2 and beta carotene (which may explain why vegetarians do better when it comes to cancer). But women especially were low on iron and vitamins B_1 and B_{12} (lack of which can cause irritability and depression). Those most at risk tended to go in for more junk foods — even though they were vegetarian. The moral seems to be to eat a good balanced diet, taking especial care to get enough vitamins and minerals. And if you do suffer any troublesome symptoms, see a nutritional specialist to see if you could benefit from a supplement.

Further details: The McCarrison Society, 23 Stanley Court, Worcester Road, Sutton, Surrey, SM2 6SD. Tel: 01 643 2812. The Vegetarian Society, 53 Marloes Road, London W8 6LA.

Your Guide to Vitamins and Minerals

A (fat soluble)
Sources: Liver, cheese, eggs, carrots, green leafy vegetables, tomatoes, dried apricots, oily fish
Why you need it: For healthy bones and teeth, better eyesight, helps resist infection, helps you resist cancer.

B$_1$ Thiamin (water soluble)
Sources: Brown rice, wholegrain cereals and breads, pork, liver, peas, seeds, nuts, molasses, Brewer's yeast
Why you need it: Helps digestion, healthy blood, muscle tone, eyes, heart, hair, brain and nervous system, and helps inhibit pain.

B$_2$ Riboflavin (water soluble)
Sources: Spinach, leafy green vegetables, eggs, wholegrains, brown rice, meat, cheese, liver, kidney, fish, molasses, Brewer's yeast
Why you need it: Fights infection, aids red blood-cell formation, helps your body process protein.

B$_6$ (water soluble)
Sources: Liver, beef, oily fish, wholegrain products, wheatgerm, walnuts, peanuts, molasses, prunes, avocados, raisins, bananas, cabbage and leafy green vegetables, carrots
Why you need it: Helps fight infection, helps your body use magnesium and linoleic acid, helps in sodium/potassium balance of body. Especially useful for a number of women's menstrual problems and those connected with menopause. Healthy blood, nerves, muscles and skin.

B$_{12}$ (water soluble)
Sources: Kidney, liver, heart, eggs, herrings, mackerel, cottage cheese
Why you need it: For cell growth, to help iron absorption, and processing of fats, carbohydrates and proteins in diet. Healthy blood and nervous systems.

Folic Acid (water soluble)
Sources: Leafy green vegetables, milk products, bananas, liver, kidney, citrus fruits, oysters
Why you need it: For healthy blood (prevents anaemia), glands and liver, helps circulation, cell growth, and stimulates appetite.

Niacin (water soluble)
Sources: Wheat and wholewheat products, peanuts, eggs, meat, fish
Why you need it: Helps circulation, helps reduce cholesterol. Healthy hair, brain, heart, and other internal organs. Aids production of sex hormones.

Pantothenic Acid (water soluble)
Sources: Liver, kidney, eggs, wheatgerm, milk, cheese, spinach, potatoes, mushrooms
Why you need it: Helps remove poisons from system. Helps body deal with stress, helps it to make use of vitamins. Healthy adrenal glands, digestive system, immune system, nerves and skin.

Vitamin C (water soluble)
Sources: Green vegetables, potatoes, citrus fruits, blackcurrants
Why you need it: Helps digestion, aids healing, prevents bleeding, helps resist coughs and colds and other infections. Healthy adrenal glands, blood, blood vessels, skin, bones, teeth and gums. Especially necessary if you smoke, drink or are under stress. Some experts claim it can help treat cancer.

D (fat soluble)
Sources: Eggs, liver, oily fish, cream, butter, cheese, sunlight
Why you need it: Helps your body utilize calcium and phosphorus important if you are to avoid osteoporosis (brittle bones) in middle age. Helps heart to pump, maintains nervous system, aids blood clotting. Healthy bones, heart, nerves, skin, teeth, thyroid.

Vitamin E (fat soluble)
Sources: Eggs, cereals, peanuts, fruit, nuts, vegetable oils, milk products
Why you need it: May delay ageing, reduces cholesterol levels in blood, improved blood flow, possible aid to fertility. Healthy blood vessels, heart, lungs, nerves, skin and pituitary function.

K (fat soluble)
Sources: Lean meat, liver, most vegetables, cereals, molasses, yogurt
Why you need it: Healthy blood, blood clotting, healthy liver function.

Calcium
Sources: Sardines, soya, milk, cheese, yogurt, watercress, molasses, nuts
Why you need it: Healthy blood, bones, teeth, skin, soft tissue, heart. Especially important for avoidance of osteoporosis (brittle bones) in middle age. Helps calm nerves, regulates heart.

Chromium
Sources: Brewer's yeast, wholegrains, liver, cheese, molasses
Why you need it: Healthy blood and circulation, helps balance blood sugar level, and regulate energy levels.

Copper
Sources: Lobster, nuts, raisins, wheatgerm, olives, molasses, avocados
Why you need it: Helps haemoglobin formation, helps regulate emotions. Healthy blood, skin, circulation, hair, bones.

Iodine
Sources: Fish, fruit, vegetables
Why you need it: Regulates thyroid activity, helps produce energy. Healthy hair, nails, skin, teeth.

Iron
Sources: Meat, liver, eggs, sardines, pulses, oats, wholemeal bread, figs, prunes, dried apricots, cocoa, molasses
Why you need it: Formation of red blood cells, helps resists stress. Healthy blood, nails, bones, skin.

Magnesium
Sources: Meat, poultry, fish, nuts, bran, milk, honey, eggs, green vegetables, wholemeal flour, brown rice, Brewer's yeast
Why you need it: Acid/alkaline balance of body, energy metabolism, aids absorption of calcium and vitamin C, may help prevent PMS (pre-menstrual-syndrome). Healthy blood vessels, heart, muscles, teeth, nerves.

Phosphorus
Sources: Meat, milk, eggs, grains, yellow cheeses
Why you need it: Bone and tooth formation, cell growth and repair, helps body use vitamins and absorb sugar and calcium. Healthy bones, brain, nerves, muscles, teeth, kidneys.

Potassium
Sources: Meat, vegetables, dates, figs, peaches, molasses, peanuts, raisins, bananas
Why you need it: Helps calm you down, controls heartbeat, muscle contraction. Healthy blood, heart, muscles, nerves, kidneys, skin.

Selenium
Sources: Eggs, fish, whole grains, brown rice, meat, poultry, nuts
Why you need it: Helps pancreas to work properly, may help fight off cancer. Healthy tissues.

Sodium
Sources: Salt, milk, cheese
Why you need it: Regulates fluid levels in cells, prevents cramp. Healthy blood, muscles, nerves, lymphatic system.

Zinc
Sources: Beef, liver, seafood, oysters, nuts, cheese, wholemeal bread, carrots, sweetcorn, tomatoes, ginger, mushrooms, sunflower seeds
Why you need it: Helps healing of wounds, helps digestion of starchy food, may help avoid anorexia (not proved), counters depression, aids metabolism of B_1, phosphorus and protein. Healthy blood and heart, healthy sex organs.

Exercise

Exercise makes you look and feel better. It puts a spring in your step and a glow in your skin. It helps keep your weight under control, reduces your chance of a heart attack, helps you sleep better, eat better and feel less depressed. It tones up your muscles and gives you more stamina. Exercise helps you cope with stress. So why don't more of us do it?

One reason perhaps is that women are brought up to think of themselves as passive and weak. Sportiness is associated with being unfeminine. And even the frenetic jogging and working-out of the current fitness craze seems to have at least as much to do with the attainment of an unrealistic female shape, as with the health benefits. What's more, if you you're unused to it, exercise hurts! Your muscles feel sore, your joints ache, and at least to begin with you feel older and even more liable to fall to pieces than ever.

However, it's well worth persevering because the right kind of exercise really can help you withstand stresses and strains more easily. The secret is to choose a form of exercise that suits you. If you enjoy it you're more likely to stick with it. There are innumerable forms of exercise to choose from. And one advantage of the fitness boom is that so many different sorts of exercise are available wherever you live. Which should you go for? Ask yourself these questions:

● How much time do I have to spare?

● How much money can I afford?

● Would I like to exercise on my own or with others?

● What's available in my area?

● What are my particular physical strengths and weaknesses?

● What sports or physical activities did I enjoy at school?

● What sports or physical activities do I enjoy watching?

If you're not the sporty type, some of the movement awareness techniques such as Yoga, T'ai Chi, Alexander Technique or dance may suit you better than taking up a sport. If you dislike the hearty image of sports there are plenty of other ways to exercise, either alone or in company.

If the social side is important to you, join a keep fit class, or gym if you can afford it. If you feel embarrassed at the thought of working-out with all those beefy chaps go for one that holds women-only sessions. Incidentally, when first starting to exercise doing it with a friend can help keep up flagging motivation when it starts to hurt, or when the fireside seems more appealing than going to your workout.

If you are busy, choose something that will fit easily into your working day, or you'll be tempted to give up. How about cycling to work? Swimming in the lunch hour? Going for a work-out immediately after you finish work?

If you've got small children you could go for an exercise that will involve them too. Local baths may hold 'duckling' sessions for toddlers. And there are several books around showing how you can exercise together. Alternatively, choose a daytime class with a crèche, if there is one in your area, or get a babysitter and get completely away for one evening a week.

If you prefer exercising alone, then, running, swimming, walking and cycling are good all-round choices.

Starting to exercise is the hardest step.

Once you've started to feel the benefits you won't want to give up.

The three main aims of exercise are to build up strength, mobility and stamina. Observe the following rules and you'll soon begin to reap the benefits of being fitter:

● Always spend some time warming up and cooling down.

● Choose an exercise you think you'll enjoy. You can use the visualization technique described on page 14 to help you decide what possibilities there might be.

● Try to exercise at least three times a week.

● Work up gradually — don't overstrain yourself. 'Going for the burn' can be positively harmful.

● Find out as much as you can about particular exercises, what parts of your body are used, whether it's aerobic (i.e. designed to increase oxygen intake and therefore energy) and so on. Then try to choose a series of exercises to provide a balance.

● If you develop physical signs such as ulcers, sore throats, sleeplessness, fatigue, you could be overdoing it. Stay in touch with your body and know when to stop.

● Exercise will often iron out period problems, but if you are suffering badly from PMS or pain it may be better to delay exercising until you feel better. A relaxation session instead may be what you need to put you in a better frame of mind. Be guided by your body. See chapter on period problems (page 47) for more suggestions.

Which exercise?

Walking
Cost: Low. You don't need any special equipment beyond a pair of good, strong shoes and something waterproof in case it rains.
Suitability: Suits all ages, and states of health. Can be fitted easily into your everyday life if you're very busy.
Advantages: Exercises your heart, burns up energy, yet is gentle and non-stressful. Helps clear your mind. Some claim to reach an almost meditative state while walking.

Swimming
Cost: Low.
Suitability: Suits all ages and levels of physical fitness. Can be useful if you suffer from a heart condition (always consult your doctor first), if you are overweight, or have arthritis. Available wherever you live.
Advantages: Good for posture. Exercises most of your major muscles including the heart. Has been called the best all-round exercise. You can pace yourself. Helps relaxation. Water is soothing, especially the sea. Good if you're pregnant as the water takes your weight.

Cycling
Cost: A good bike can be fairly expensive, but it's a once-only expenditure. If you plan to take up cycling seriously you may want to join a club and buy special clothing (which will increase costs).
Suitability: Good for any age. If you have children you can all cycle together.
Advantages: Once you've learned the basics you can cycle almost anywhere, though town cycling is not always pleasant or safe. Good for your heart and lower limbs. Doesn't do a lot for your upper body. Good way of meeting people if you join a club. Risks of back injury, heat and cold. Wear correct clothing, and pay attention to how you ride.

Dance
Cost: Varies according to where you go and type of dance you choose. Leotards, tights, and so on can all mount up.
Suitability: Anyone of any age or state of fitness can do it. Women especially often feel a real affinity for dance as a form. Find out about different types, for instance belly dancing is a wonderful, sensuous form of dance especially suited to women — even a round stomach is an advantage!
Advantages: Allows you to express emotions in movement. Increases flexiblity, develops leg muscles. Good way to meet others. Some types of dance likely to be available wherever you live.

Running/Jogging
Cost: Cheap, though running shoes can be expensive and you should go for the best you can afford.
Suitability: Any age, you can do it anywhere, anytime which makes it specially useful if you're busy and don't have much time.
Advantages: Exercises your heart and lungs, and legs. Good for meeting people if that's what you want, or you can do it alone. Runners 'high' releases endorphins into system giving sense of well-being.

Of course these are just a few of the exercises you can take up. **For further ideas** see:
Fit for the Future: The guide for women who want to live well, Jeanette Winterson, (Pandora).
The Active Woman's Health Guide, Dr Wendy Dodds and Paul Wade (Breslich and Foss).

Exercise in pregnancy
Exercise in pregnancy can build up your strength and suppleness so you are better able to cope with the extra demands on your body. It can also help you cope better with labour — though it can't guarantee you an easy birth. It helps you relax and combat sleeping problems, and gives you a feeling of well-being. Dance is an especially suitable form of exercise if you are pregnant. At St George's Hospital, London, they even employ a dance therapist to hold classes for mums-to-be. Follow these guidelines for safe exercise in pregnancy.

● Check with your medical advisor before embarking on an exercise routine.

● If you're not used to exercising go gently, and stop if you feel any pain.

● Don't make yourself feel worn out.

● Go for non-weight-bearing exercising

such as swimming, cycling or types of stretching which doesn't have bouncing actions. Ease off exercise other than stretching in the last four weeks.

● Avoid surfing, windsurfing, mountain climbing, skydiving and other dangerous activities. Sport or exercises involving precise balance and co-ordination may be more risky as your centre of gravity changes and your sense of balance may be affected.

● Exercise regularly so long as pregnancy is straightforward — but no sudden bursts.

● Exercise for shorter periods and take regular rests, in order to maintain blood supply to the baby.

● Take your pulse every 10 to 15 minutes. If it rises to 140 a minute slow down until it is 90 or under.

● Don't get too hot. If your baby gets overheated it can cause problems, especially during the first three months. Avoid exercising for longer than half an hour at a time, if it's hot or muggy.

● Cut down on hot baths and saunas.

● Rest for 10 minutes lying on your left side after exercise to allow your body to recover.

● Drink two or three glasses of water after

exercising to replace fluids lost through sweating. Drink whenever you feel thirsty during exercise.

● Increase the amount you eat to replace calories burnt off by exercise.

● Stop exercising straight away if you get out of breath, feel dizzy, numb, experience pins and needles, pain or bleeding. Consult your doctor.

For further information:
Weight Control in Pregnancy by Dr Jennifer J. Ashcroft and Dr R. Glynn Owens, (Thorsons).
Swimming Through Your Pregnancy by Jane Katz, (Thorsons).

Don't neglect your pelvic floor

Your pelvic floor is the hammock of muscle that lies between your pubic bone and your lower spine. The muscles form a figure eight around the bladder, uterus and bowel and hold them in place. You use them when you are making love to squeeze your partner's penis or fingers, during childbirth to allow the baby to emerge smoothly, and to control the flow of urine.

Sometimes the muscles can become slack and flabby. This can be a result of too little exercise, too hard pushing during childbirth, overweight, a job that involves a lot of heavy lifting, and simply age, which reduces the amount of oestrogen in your system. If you lose tone in your pelvic floor you may suffer any or all of the following:

● a floppy vagina with less sensation

● prolapse of the uterus (when your uterus drops out of place)

● inability to fully empty your bladder, leading to increased urine infections

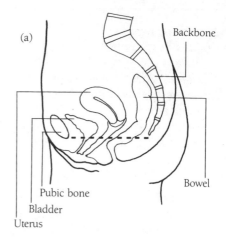

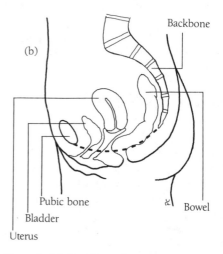

Figure 2: (a) Position of organs in the body with good pelvic floor support.
(b) With poor support the organs descend and the pelvic floor sags.

● constipation

● stress incontinence, i.e. leaking of urine if you laugh, sneeze, cough or run around

● fatigue on standing for too long, and a heavy dragging feeling as if your 'insides are falling out'.

Fortunately, it's possible to improve your pelvic floor muscles at any age. The secret is pelvic-floor exercises, (sometimes called Kegel exercises). These are invisible exercises that you can perform any time of day, when you are talking on the phone, waiting in a bus queue or whatever. They involve tightening and lifting the pelvic floor.

Identify the muscles by trying to stop the flow of urine. If the muscles are weak you may have some trouble doing this. Don't persist until you have built up some strength as you may weaken them even further. You can also identify the muscles by trying to grip one or two fingers placed in your vagina, either your own or your partner's, or your partner's penis. If your muscles are strong your partners will wince with pleasure . . . this is known as positive feedback! Don't worry if contractions get weaker as you continue squeezing — it's perfectly normal.

The exercises
1. Tighten up the whole pelvic floor and hold it for three seconds, relax. Repeat five times. Do this several times a day, working up gradually until you are doing about 10 sets of these exercises a day. If your muscles feel sore, step down the number of exercises temporarily to allow them to recover.
2. Childbirth expert Sheila Kitzinger calls this the 'invisible lift'. Imagine your pelvic floor is a lift, gradually raise it to the first, second, third, fourth and fifth floors stopping briefly on each one. Then go down again gradually. Always tighten your pelvic floor at the end of this exercise. After all you wouldn't walk around with your mouth hanging open would you, so why do it with your pelvic floor?
3. Draw up and relax your pelvic floor

quickly, as though pumping water in and out of your vagina.

Don't overstrain yourself, and work up gradually. And always remember to tighten your muscles at the end of each exercise.

Benefits of looking after your pelvic floor
● a better sex life

● helps your body cope better with the stress and strain of pregnancy and birth

● helps avoid stress incontinence

Incidentally there's evidence from a study carried out at Northwick Park Hospital that *any* exercise, not just those aimed specifically at this area, can improve pelvic floor tone.

If you do suffer from a weak pelvic floor, osteopathy may be able to help, by correcting imbalances in posture that may have affected the muscular hammock. Yoga exercises are also beneficial, and you'll find several suitable ones in *Yoga and Pregnancy* by Sophy Hoare, (Unwin).

Finally, your pelvic floor may be weakened if you have a persistent cough, so try to get this cleared up. Avoid constipation by eating a high fibre diet. And if you are experiencing pelvic floor symptoms such as those mentioned earlier, which don't go away despite a concentrated programme of pelvic-floor exercises, see your doctor, as you may need surgery, or treatment such as a special ring pessary to support the uterus.

Looking after your body

Your breasts
Many of us feel discontented with our breasts. We feel they're too small (usually) or (more rarely) too big. This is hardly

surprising given the fact that a pair of boobs draped over a sports car can be used to sell almost anything. Becoming familiar with our breasts can help us learn to like them, and accept them as part of ourselves whether they are firm or soft, big or small. Examining your breasts can also help you detect any small changes that may be a sign of cancer or benign breast disease at an early stage.

Advantages of examining your breasts:

● You become familiar with what they feel like at different stages of your cycle

● Nine out of ten breast lumps are discovered by women during self examination

When should you do it? Your breasts will be easier to examine and less lumpy immediately after your period.

How to do it

1. Stand in front of a mirror with your arms by your side and look at your breasts. You're looking for any changes in texture such as dimpling or an orange peel appearance. There's a wide variation in women's breasts. If you've had a baby, been on the pill or lost a lot of weight you may be able to see little silvery ridges that are stretch marks.
2. Next lie down. Place a cushion or towel under your shoulder and feel firmly but gently. A circular motion is best, moving from breast bone to the nipple, around it and under your arms. If you're unsure how to do it, ask a doctor or nurse, at the family planning clinic for example, to show you how. Make sure that you examine each part of your breast.
3. Repeat on the other side.

What you are looking for

Any changes on the surface of your skin or deeper lumps. Most lumps turn out to be harmless. A fluid-filled mass that feels like a peeled grape will usually be a cyst, a fatty tumour that hurts when you squeeze may be a fibroadenoma. The sort of lump to be most suspicious of is a hard mass that doesn't move, seems to grow into the surrounding tissue or be anchored to the chest wall.

If you *find* any sort of lump, though, you should see your doctor, to put your mind at rest.

To screen or not to screen

Conventional wisdom says we should each examine our breasts every month. However, unless you've been taught how to examine

Figure 3.

Breast self-examination.

(a) Look at yourself in a mirror.

(b) Put your hands on your head and look for any irregularities, especially around the nipples.

(c) Stretch your arms above your head and look again.

(d) repeat procedure, this time with your hands on your hips.

(e) Lie on a flat surface with your shoulder slightly raised by a towel. Feel your left breast with your right hand, using the flat part of your fingers.

(f) Working in a circle, feel every part of your breast.

(g) With your left arm behind your head, repeat the circular movement, especially around the outer part of the breast.

(h) Finish by feeling the tail of the breast towards the armpit. Repeat with the other beast.

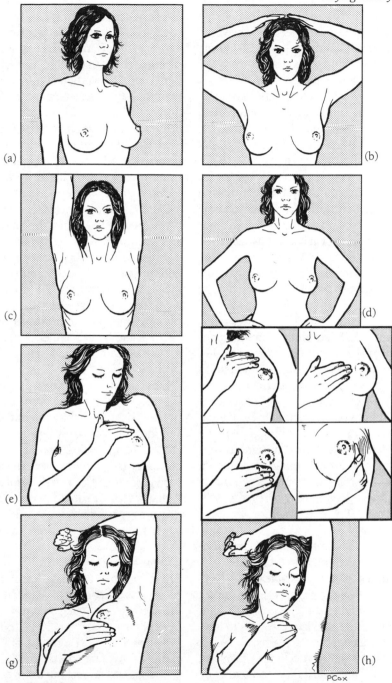

(a)

(b)

(c)

(d)

(e)

(f)

(g)

(h)

Figure 3

yourself properly there's no guarantee that you will detect a lump earlier than you would through casual handling. In the meantime you may have subjected yourself to a process which has made you extremely anxious.

Massive health education campaigns to get us all to examine ourselves have been singularly unsuccessful. Why? One expert writing in a medical magazine points out that psychologically, breast self examination is not very satisfying: the 'reward' you get for doing it is the discovery that you have a serious, and sometimes fatal disease. Some authorities point out that by the time a lump is large enough to be felt it will usually have been there sometime. What's more, some large lumps are very slow growing, while some small ones are of an aggressive type that gets worse very quickly.

So what should you do? The answer seems to be that if you feel secure by examining your breasts, go ahead and do it. On the other hand, if the whole process distresses you and you decide not to do it, you aren't necessarily reducing your chances of successful treatment if you do get cancer since chances are you will discover any lumps there are to be felt when you wash or handle your breasts in the normal course of events. At present large trials are being carried out to assess the effectiveness of breast self-examination (BSE).

Mammography
Screening with mammography (a breast X-ray) can detect a lump before it is big enough to feel. It's not widely available on the NHS purely as a screening method, though it's frequently used to aid diagnosis. A slight disadvantage is that it exposes you to low-doses of radiation, in itself a risk of breast cancer. However, if you fall into a high risk group — for instance if there is a tendency

to breast cancer in your family — you will need to balance up the relative risks.

A Scandinavian study has shown that deaths from breast cancer have fallen by 31 per cent in women who were given mammographic screening. An interim report from a massive British study being carried out in Edinburgh has shown that slow growing tumours are more frequently detected at a first screening, and a higher proportion of the more aggressive, fast growing cancers at subsequent screenings.

Mammography appears to be most useful if you are over 50, when the amount of fat and glandular tissue in the breasts makes it easier to detect any abnormalities. The denser breast tissue of younger women makes mammography less useful, though a new technique called 'light scanning' (dia-phanoscopy) which involves a very bright beam being shone into the breast is claiming a 90 per cent success rate in detecting cancers.

It has to be said that breast cancer death is caused by the spread of the cancer cells (metastasis) rather than the initial tumour. This doesn't necessarily depend on the size of the initial lump. So spending vast amounts of money on detecting ever smaller lumps is no guarantee of more successful treatment. Perhaps what we should be doing is looking to more ways of preventing cancer, and this is where alternative health care can come in.

'Down below'

There's one part of our bodies about which most of us are completely ignorant, despite the fact it plays such an important and fundamental part in our lives — our genitals. We allow our most intimate orifices to be explored by our lovers, or the doctor's rubber-gloved fingers, but the majority of us

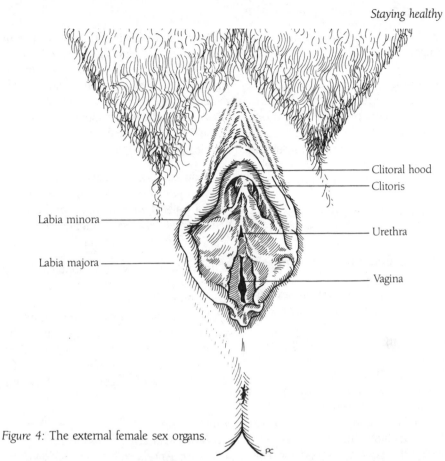

Labia minora

Labia majora

Clitoral hood

Clitoris

Urethra

Vagina

Figure 4: The external female sex organs.

have no idea what we look like 'down below'.

Getting familiar with this part of your body can be an important part of getting to know yourself. Each of us is different, just as the noses on our faces are all different. It can remove the mystery from our genitals and help us feel more at ease with our sexuality. It can help you spot any potential health problem, such as an erosion or infection, at an early stage, so that you can begin treatment or seek help. You will be able to detect any changes earlier than a doctor who only examines you occasionally. It can help you take control of your own fertility by practising natural family planning methods.

Some women examine themselves together with other women in a women's health group, as part of the process of demystifying health care and getting to know their own bodies. But there's no reason why you shouldn't examine yourself at home.

What you will need

● a torch or Anglepoise type lamp

● a mirror

● a plastic speculum — this is the 'beak' like instrument doctors use to do an internal. You can buy one from the Women's Health Information Centre (address on page 37) or your local women's group or women's health group might sell them.

What you can expect to see

1. Start by examining your outer genitals. You'll see the fatty pad called the 'mons veneris' covered by pubic hair. In some women this can extend some way up the abdomen, and down onto their thighs. The hair covers the outer lips of your genitals — the labia majora.
2. Next, using the mirror if necessary, explore between the outer lips. You'll see the inner lips (labia minora). These can be anything from pinkish to purplish-brown in colour, and may look thin and ragged or plump. When you are sexually aroused they become swollen, increasing sensation.

   At the top inside your inner lips you'll find your clitoris. It's a small pink 'button' partly covered by a hood of skin, and is exquisitely sensitive. In fact it's the heart of women's sexual arousal.

   Spread the inner lips and you will see next to your clitoris the urinary opening, and below that your vaginal opening. This is normally closed, but stretches and fans out like a flower during sexual arousal or childbirth. If you are a virgin and have never used tampons you may find the vagina covered in a thin membrane called the hymen.
3. Now you're ready to look inside your vagina. Insert the speculum gently and lock it open. You'll see your cervix or neck of the womb, like a shiny rosy knob with a dimple in the middle — the *os*. If you've had children this will be slightly wider. You'll notice your vaginal secretions, and will be able to tell if you have an infection (see page 65).

● If you see a reddened shiny area on your cervix, this is probably an erosion. This can be caused by a variety of factors — being on the Pill, recent childbirth, irritation from an IUD (coil), or hormone imbalance. In most cases it will go without treatment, but it would be wise to see the doctor for a check up. (See also page 74.)

● If you examine yourself at different times in your cycle you'll notice your cervix and vaginal walls change in colour and texture. Your cervix also gets higher or lower depending on where you are in your cycle.

● It's best not to examine yourself during pregnancy. Once you've tried self-examination you may want to make it a regular part of your health care routine, or you may feel satisfied to leave it to the medics. But whether you do it once or adopt self-examination as a regular practice, it can be an enormously enlightening and exciting experience.

Further information:
Our Bodies, Ourselves, A Healthy Book by and for Women, Angela Phillips and Jill Rakusen, (Penguin).
For Ourselves, Our bodies and sexuality — from women's point of view, Anja Meulenbelt, (Sheba).

Self help health care groups

Many women in various parts of the country have set up self help health groups. The idea is to share information and experiences, to demystify health care, and to provide a different way of looking at health care and caring for our bodies.

Such a health group may be held in someone's home, a women's centre, health or community centre.

The Women's Health Information Centre has information about groups throughout the country, or you might be interested in forming one of your own. Activities and subjects that might be included are:

- Self-examination
- Periods and their problems
- Birth control
- Childbirth
- Sexuality
- Cancer
- The menopause
- Alternative therapies.

Above all such groups are positive and practical.

Further information:
Women's Health Information Centre, 52/54 Featherstone Street, London EC1.

Smoking

Lung cancer seems all set to replace breast cancer as number one cancer killer for women. Smoking is strongly linked with cancer of the cervix. If you take the Pill and smoke you have a three times higher risk than normal of getting heart disease. Smoking has been associated with early menopause. And if you smoke while you are expecting a baby, you're more likely to suffer a miscarriage, give birth to a low birth-weight baby, and experience problems during pregnancy and labour.

Barriers to giving it up
Anti-smoking propaganda is a classic bit of victim blaming — it's *your* fault if you smoke and it serves you right if you get any of the diseases I've already mentioned. The finger of blame is especially pointed at mums-to-be who smoke. But all this condemnation ignores one fact — the reason why people smoke in the first place. Research shows that women have special difficulties in giving up. Why?

Lighting up a cigarette can be a safety valve. It helps you calm down and reduces tension that you feel you can't get rid of in any other way. One woman quoted in a book on women's health says: 'If a bloke's fed up he can walk out of the door. You can't because of the kids and so you light up a cigarette.'

Another woman in the *The Ladykillers: Why Smoking is a Feminist Issue*, Barbara Jacobson, (Pluto) a study of women smokers says: 'I don't want to scream and yell and hurt people so I smoke.'

What's more, those around us can actively sabotage our efforts to stop. If we are ratty or irritable it isn't unknown for a member of the family to pop out for a packet of fags, 'To stop Mum being bad-tempered.'

Having a cigarette is also a way of breaking up the day, or relieving boredom. Women who are anxious, worried or depressed, or who are in stressful jobs, smoke for similar reasons.

A big barrier to giving up for many women is the fear of putting on weight. Smoking calms the appetite and can be a non-fattening alternative to a visit to the biscuit box.

A point made in a leaflet published by the

Giving it up

● Eating more fresh fruit and vegetables helps you give up smoking, according to a study from the Department of Psychology at New Columbia University. Apparently fruit and vegetables make the body more alkaline, thus making it expel nicotine more slowly, and by reducing the rate at which nicotine leaves your body, extends the time before you need your next 'fix'.

● Take up exercise. As we've already seen exercise releases endorphins, giving you a sense of well being that may reduce the nicotine craving.

● Join a self help group, or give up smoking with a friend or partner.

● Hypnosis and acupuncture can both be beneficial; hypnosis by its relaxation effect, and acupuncture by its endorphin-releasing quality. But, as an acupuncturist warned me, 'It can't enable someone to give up if they don't really want to.'

● Learn to relax. (See page 44.) But relaxation on its own isn't enough. Smoking is not just a chemical addiction, it's also to do with the way you live. Work out the times when you feel the need to smoke and plan ahead so as to avoid or cope with them. The stress reduction techniques outlined below will come in handy here. Simply learning how to view a stressful situation in a different light may help. Psychotherapy which uses 'cognitive restructuring' techniques (i.e. changing the way you think) can be useful here.

● Alter your routine. Take up knitting, join a group, read a book, play with worry beads . . . anything to take your mind off the dread weed.

● Avoid smoky places and atmospheres as well as situations in which you would normally smoke.

Women's Health Information Centre, is that many women find it hard to stop because we're not brought up to focus on long term goals. Much of our lives consists of filling in time in the short term: waiting to get married, to have a family, for the kids to grow up, the phone to ring. This particularly relates to the fear of getting fat if we give up smoking: 'The effect that excess weight will have on her life and self-image can seem a greater threat than contracting a disabling disease many years in the future.'

Much of cigarette advertising is aimed at women, with smoking being portrayed as sophisticated and glamorous.

Understanding the reasons why *you* smoke can enable you to develop strategies that will help you give up. And once you have done so you will feel and be a lot healthier.

Stress

It may seem odd to include stress in a chapter on how to stay well. Nonetheless, learning how to deal with stress is one of the most important ways in which we can help ourselves to stay healthy. And with increasing research it looks like being the linking point between alternative and orthodox approaches, and may well turn out to be the key to how and why so many of the alternative therapies work.

There's hardly an illness in existence that doesn't involve a large dose of stress. Indeed many alternative practitioners and not a few orthodox ones would claim that stress lies at the root of most ailments. Even so, stress is an inescapable part of life. As stress expert Hans Selye has said, 'Complete freedom from stress is death.' It's worth bearing this in mind since we so often think of stress as an entirely bad thing. A certain amount of stress give us the get-up-and-go necessary for living. It can also be a useful pointer. It can provide the impetus for change and give us the motivation and insight into things that are bothering us so that we can take action. That said, severe, prolonged stress is dangerous. It affects every system of our bodies and can lead to serious illness.

Women's lives, women's stress

Sources of stress come from outside and from within. Living in today's world we are exposed to noise, pollution, traffic, over-crowding. At the same time, we often feel isolated, trapped in our own homes, without the intimate relationships that can support us and sustain us in the face of day to day difficulties. Of course, most of these outside stress factors affect men too, but women are exposed to additional effects of these stressors by virtue of living in a man's world.

If you are a mother with small children you have to face the daily aggravation of living in a world where children are at best tolerated as a nuisance, at worst totally ignored. Try struggling to the shops with a baby or toddler in tow fighting your way through swing doors too narrow for a pushchair, not to mention the hassle of public transport for starters.

If you go out to work you may have had to face barriers to getting the sort of job you want, lack of training opportunities and discriminatory attitudes. You may have to work part-time, in a badly paid job with unsociable hours because of lack of training or because it's the only one that fits in with family commitments.

If you're trying to juggle home and work there are even more stresses. Women are the ones who overwhelmingly make and maintain childcare arrangements. You're probably knocking yourself out to prove you're as good as the next one at work, then rushing off home to cater for the family. Despite ideas of equality old habits die hard and women still carry the main burden of looking after home and family. Lack of official recognition of the needs of families, limited childcare facilities, subtle and not so subtle pressure to conform to certain images of womanhood can all make us feel guilty about working outside the home at all. This is despite the fact that four times as many families would be below the poverty line were it not for wives' wages. The stereotype of the high-powered career woman, who puts the demands of the board-meeting before the needs of her children, serves to perpetuate and obscure the real issues. And it all adds up to further stress.

When you add on the stresses connected with the biological milestones that punctuate our lives — menstruation, pregnancy, menopause, — it's hardly surprising so many of us fall prey to stress related disorders.

The message put across by doctors, the media, employers and others around us is that everyone should be stable and rational at all times. If we are not we risk being labelled 'ill' or in need of treatment. Perhaps the fact that nine out of ten of us suffer mood changes connected with our menstrual cycles should prompt the questions 'What is normal?' and 'Who says?'.

Nonetheless, the interaction of such social, psychological and biological factors in the face of expectations of others add up to a big stress potential. Large numbers of us feel, and in fact have, little control over our lives. And for many of us stress is long-term. It's these two factors — lack of control and prolonged stress — that experts believe are so debilitating to health.

Under stress

What happens when you are under stress? Quite simply the body prepares to cope with the threat to its equilibrium by the familiar 'fight' or 'flight' mechanism. In physical terms the hormones adrenaline and noradrenaline are released into the bloodstream, causing the following:

● Your heart beats faster

● Your blood pressure rises

● Your breathing gets faster and lighter

● Your muscles tighten ready for action

● Your mouth becomes dry (saliva dries up)

● Your digestive system closes down so that blood can be diverted to other parts of the body

● Your pupils get bigger

● Your liver releases sugar into the system to give you extra energy

● Your urine output is affected as a result of blood flow to the kidneys being reduced

● Your immune system shuts down

It's hardly surprising, where the body is under continual stress, that these powerful effects can taken their toll on your health. The physical effects of stress have a knock-on effect if they go on for any length of time — high blood-pressure can lead to heart problems, constant release of acids into the stomach leads to stomach problems such as colitis, irritable bowel, diverticulitis, ulcers and so on, and when the immune system closes down, your body is less able to deal with infection.

Are you under stress?
Tick any symptoms you regularly experience.

☐ Headaches

☐ Dry mouth

☐ Sweaty palms

☐ Dizziness

☐ Rashes

☐ Panic attacks or anxiety

☐ Problems relaxing

☐ Mind constantly on-the-go

☐ Yawning or sighing

☐ Swallowing difficulties

☐ Palpitations

☐ Sexual problems

☐ Indigestion

☐ Irritable bowel

☐ Menstrual problem

☐ Bursting into tears

☐ Aches and pains in the muscles e.g. your shoulders, back, stomach

☐ Excessive drinking or smoking

☐ Loss of appetite

☐ Compulsive eating

☐ Exhaustion even after a good night's sleep

☐ Sleeping difficulties — either sleeping too little or too much

☐ Lack of concentration

☐ Irritability

☐ Anxiety about your health

☐ Muscle twitches

☐ Low self esteem

☐ Lack of concentration

☐ Loss of interest in life

☐ Cold hands and feet (through poor circulation)

Adding up the stress factors

Psychologists Thomas Holmes and Richard Rahe discovered a link between the number of stressful events in your life and emotional and physical health. To assess this, they developed a stress scale. You can see an adaptation of it on page 42. How does your life add up?

Useful though it is, there are one or two points worth bearing in mind about this scale. The scale reflects dominant social values such as the importance of marriage as a source of stability. In fact marriage itself can be a source of stress and ill health for women. And though there's no denying the pressures on women when a relationship has broken down, often linked with the material disadvantages they suffer, research has shown that single women are far healthier than single men, and that married women are unhealthier than married men.

Women may be especially at risk of stress from relationship breakdown because for many of us our identity is tied up with other people. Try writing down ten sentences beginning with the words 'I am. :' and see how many of them relate to you as an appendage of the others in your life.

Secondly it's hard to disentangle the effects of stress such as increased smoking, drinking, poor eating habits, and all the habits that we may adopt in an effort to cope with stress, from the stress itself. And as you'll see in the rest of the book, these in themselves can affect our ability to withstand disease.

Finally, if you're worried or upset you may be more inclined to visit the doctor with symptoms that you might otherwise ignore. Women often find it especially hard to ask for help, and visiting the doctor can be a way of getting the nurture and attention you feel unable to ask for any other way.

That said there's no doubt that stressful events do play a role in illness. For instance, a study in the USA found that the husbands of women who had recently died of breast cancer had severely lowered immune response for some time afterwards. Looking at the stress scale it's not hard to see how a cascade of stress can occur. Take a pregnancy for example. Chances are this will lead on to changes in your sex life, your financial state, your working habits, job, sleep, eating habits and quite a few others. The point is it all adds up to stress.

Working out your stress score

In the last year have you experienced:

Death of your partner	100	Change in responsibilities at work	29
Divorce	73		
Marital separation	65	Children leaving home	29
Jail-term	63	Trouble with in-laws	29
Death of close family member	63	Outstanding personal achievement	28
Personal injury or illness	53		
Marriage	50	Spouse begins or stops work	26
Fired from your job	47	Begin or end school	26
Marital reconciliation	45	Change in living conditions	25
Retirement	45	Change of personal habits	24
Change in health of a member of your family	44	Trouble with your boss	23
		Change in working hours or conditions	20
Pregnancy	40		
Sex problems	39	House move	20
New family member	39	Change in schools	20
Business readjustment	39	Change in leisure	19
Change in financial state	38	Change in church-going habits	19
Death of close friend	37	Change in social life	18
Change to different line of work	36	Medium mortgage or loan	17
		Change in sleeping habits	16
Change in number of arguments with your partner	35	Change in number of family get-togethers	15
Large mortgage	31	Holiday	13
Foreclosure of mortgage or loan	30	Christmas	12

Score over 300 and you stand an 80 per cent chance of going down with a physical illness in the next year.

How can you help yourself?

A large part of this book boils down to helping yourself to deal with the effects of stress. So what can you do? Experts in stress reduction say a two-fold approach is most helpful:

1. Anticipate stress.
2. Develop a battery of coping strategies to help you cope with unavoidable stress.

Let's take pregnancy as an example again. Though motherhood is held up as the highest achievement we can reach, it's also downgraded in the status stakes. Anticipating stress can mean writing down all your fears and worries about becoming a mother, however trivial, and using your list as a basis for discussion and action. If you are worried about birth, for instance, you can make it your business to find out about local hospital policies and methods of pain relief, get information on how to help yourself, and book in for a course of antenatal classes. This last will put you in contact with others undergoing the same experience — a valuable counter to stress. A similar action plan can be useful for any stressful situation.

Another useful technique is 'noticing'. Instead of being waylaid by all the thoughts and feelings that fill your mind, make a point of paying attention to what is going on around you. Concentrate on your physical surrounding, the process of doing whatever you are engaged in at that moment, and so on, so as to be truly aware.

Coping with Stress

● Expect change and accept it as normal

● Don't hang on to the past

● Accept yourself as you are

● Don't do something just because you feel it is expected of you

● Learn how to say 'no'

● If you have a problem, talk about it

● Find something absorbing to do — work or a leisure activity, anything that engages your whole attention

---

● Give yourself a break. Spend time doing nothing, reading, walking, having a bath, anything you enjoy

● Hang on to your sense of humour — it really is the best medicine

● Get some exercise — physical activity releases stored up tension

● Learn to relax

● *Don't* drink more, smoke more, or take drugs

Basically what this all boils down to is looking after yourself — something women often find hard to do.

Alternative therapies
Virtually all the alternative therapies can help you deal with stress. The key is to find the one that suits you. Going to see an alternative practitioner can be something you are able to do for yourself, and can improve self esteem. It can also give you the energy to deal with stressful situations.

Psychotheraphy, co-counselling and other mind-body therapies can help identify the roots of problems. They can allow you to express emotions such as anger, fear and sorrow safely without the consequences they might have in real life.

Meditation, yoga and T'ai chi can help you relax and slow down your body and mind, giving a break from problems and reducing the harmful bodily effects listed earlier. In fact, in a study carried out at the University of Arkansas College of Medicine, meditation was shown to have a direct effect on the immune response mechanism.

Learning to relax is something positive you

can do for yourself. Anyone can do it, and you don't need special equipment.

1. Choose a time when you know you won't be interrupted, and take the phone off the hook.
2. Loosen any tight clothing, then sit or lie down.
3. Tighten each muscle in turn, working from the toes to the top of the head.
4. Now loosen each muscle, letting each one become as floppy as you can and feeling your body become heavy.
5. Stay like this for 10 to 15 minutes, breathing slowly and calmly. If any disturbing thoughts occur, as they will, simply let them flow in and out of your mind. It can help to focus your mind on a soothing scene, or concentrate on your breathing or heartbeat.

With practice you will be able to relax easily any time you want. Practise relaxation once or twice a day, and use the routine whenever you need to calm yourself during the day, for instance if you have a difficult meeting, exam or whatever.

Further information: Relaxation for Living, Dunesk, 29 Burwood Park Road, Walton on Thames, Surrey, KT12 5LH.

Learn to assert yourself
Many of us have particular difficulties in asserting ourselves and find ourselves doing things we don't really want to, or living up to other people's expectations of us instead of our own. It often arises out of the 'good girl' syndrome, in which we spend our lives trying to please other people in order to be liked. Learning to say 'no' calmly and to ask for what you want without getting upset or feeling guilty is the essence of assertiveness training. It can help give a sense of greater control over your life, which leads to a reduction in stress.

The secret of saying 'no' without feeling guilty is to acknowledge certain basic human rights. These include the right to be treated as an intelligent, capable and equal human being, to change your mind, to express your own opinions even when they conflict with those of other people, to ask other people to meet our needs and to decide whether or not to respond to theirs. Can you think of any others? Recognizing your own rights involves acknowledging those of others too, of course. And it doesn't mean getting your own way all the time. Flexibility and being able to see another's viewpoint are also important.

Being assertive doesn't mean being aggressive or unreasonable. It means being able to ask for what you want calmly and honestly without becoming angry or upset and with respect for others.

Assertive skills can be useful in all sorts of everyday situations, and also in more specific ones like during childbirth, or in dealing with the medical profession, or your partner. The techniques are simple to learn, though you'll probably learn better in a group where you can practice rather than from a book.

Further information
Many LEAs offer assertiveness courses. Contact your local adult education organizer to see if there is one in your area.
The Women's Therapy Centre, 6 Manor Gardens, London N7, offers regular women-only courses.
A useful book is *A Woman in Your Own Right*, Anne Dickson, (Quartet).

Breathing
Hyperventilation or overbreathing is the cause of many problems. Shallow, fast

breathing is a result of stress and can also increase anxious feelings. Learning to breathe slowly and calmly can help reduce tension and make you feel more energetic.

1. Sit or lie in a relaxed position.
2. Place a hand on your upper chest and one on your stomach.
3. Breathe in slowly until your bottom hand rises. If you're doing it properly the upper hand should barely move.
4. Hold your breath for a count of five, then slowly breathe out. Pause then repeat again.
5. Repeat ten times.

You can use this exercise to calm yourself if you are feeling tense, to get to sleep, or before practising meditation or relaxation.

Sleep

Anxiety can be the biggest reason for not being able to drop off at night, or perhaps you are suffering pain from a chronic illness.

● Start to wind down a couple of hours before bedtime. Read a book, practise your yoga or meditation.

● Avoid stimulating discussions or arguments.

● Have a warm bath. Add aromatic oils such as lavender, camomile, marjoram, clary sage, rose, ylang ylang.

● Get a partner or friend to give you a massage.

● Drink a herb tea such as valerian or camomile to calm your nerves. You can buy special mixtures from the health food shop such as Quiet Life which is a combination of relaxing herbs.

● Use a herb pillow.

● Listen to a relaxation tape or play a favourite piece of music.

● Avoid eating too late at night, and avoid coffee, tea, alcohol or other stimulants.

● If you can't get off, spend the time 'drifting', practising visualization or meditating to refresh and revive you. Experts think that we only need about 5 or 6 hours sleep anyway, and the odd broken night never hurt anyone in the long run. You'll be better able to withstand it if you have spent the sleepless hours relaxing.

● Above all don't panic, and try to avoid tranquillizers and sleeping pills.

Avoiding Work Stress

● Pay attention to lighting. The best type of lighting is that which is comfortable for the job.

● Don't sit for too long, — it can hamper circulation. If you can, get up and walk around ever hour or so, otherwise tap your feet.

● Pay attention to your seating. If the seating is too high, use a foot rest or a pile of books to raise it to a comfortable height.

● Don't stand for too long

- If you work with a VDU make sure you have regular breaks, and don't work on one for too long, especially if you are pregnant.

- Make sure there is adequate fresh air. Plants, flowers and bowls of water will moisten the air. An air ionizer will reduce stuffiness.

- Develop assertive skills to deal with your superiors

Of course there's not always a lot you can do on an individual level about poor working conditions. Working together with others will help.

Contact the Women and Work Hazards Groups, for further details of hazards that can affect your health at work, c/o A Woman's Place, Hungerford House, Victoria Embankment, London WC2N 6PA.

Further information
The Book of Stress Survival, Alix Kirsta, (Allen & Unwin.)
Coping with stress: a practical self-help guide for women, Georgia Witkin-Lanoil, (Sheldon Press).

PART TWO

Women's illnesses

Periods and their problems

Forty out of every thousand of us visiting the doctor each year go with period problems, and many more simply suffer in silence. Not many of us believe nowadays that we'll turn the milk sour, make bees die, rust iron or brass or stop the bread from rising when we have our periods! But all too many of us are ignorant about just what is normal, which makes it hard to know when and where to seek help.

What's normal?

One way to become familiar with your own individual pattern is to keep a menstrual diary. The variation in 'normal' is enormous and the 28-day cycle is a bit of a myth. Most of us in fact experience irregularities in cycle length, amount of bleeding and so on from time to time throughout our lives. Many period problems that have no apparent cause result from stress interfering with hormone balance. This chapter looks at what period problems you might experience and what you can do about them. However, do bear in mind that most alternative therapists don't look at symptoms in isolation, and so will probably not use the conventional classification outlined here.

Lack of periods (amenorrhoea)

The most common reasons for not having periods of course are if you are pregnant or breast-feeding. Doctors conventionally define two types of amenorrhoea: primary, when your periods have never started at all, and secondary when they have been apparently normal and then stop. In practice, the boundaries between these two are not that clear cut. Given the enormous range in cycles in those of us who are perfectly healthy, unless your symptoms are especially marked and/or you are trying to conceive there may be no need to seek help.

When to seek help

If you haven't started your periods by the time you are 18 you may need special tests to see what is causing the delay. Quite often the reason is stress or other emotional upsets. Very occasionally amenorrhoea is a result of congenital abnormalities for which, sadly, little can be done by orthodox or alternative medicine. In this, extremely unlikely, event there will usually be several other signs that something is wrong.

Hormonal disturbances affecting the thyroid, extreme weight loss (for instance if you are anorexic), drugs such as those used to treat high blood-pressure or cancer, coming off the pill, and a few rare diseases such as pituitary tumours are the most common medical reasons for lack of periods.

Conventional treatment
Conventional treatment consists of tests to find out why you aren't having periods, plus hormone treatment or drugs to stimulate the hormone producing centres in the brain, such as Clomid, a drug used to treat infertility. Very occasionally, if the cause is thought to be psychological you may be offered tranquillizers or anti-depressants.

Alternative treatment and self help
Herbal treatment is extremely effective for amenorrhoea, though a qualified herbalist advises against treating yourself. Garden sage (salvia officinalis) is useful in regulating your periods. A number of herbs can be used to rebalance your hormones, where this seems to be the underlying reason for the problem. Chaste Tree also known as Monk's Pepper (*vitex agnus castus*) is particularly useful.

Homoeopathy is a useful first line of treatment, where there are no obvious physical causes. If you are using alternative therapy and are not trying to conceive make sure you are using contraception, since if you suddenly ovulate you could become pregnant. Acupuncture is also useful.

For stress relief try biofeedback, meditation, plus the stress coping measures outlined in the previous section.

Since amenorrhoea is so tied up with infertility, you'll find further details of alternative approaches in the section dealing with fertility and reproduction.

Heavy periods (menorrhagia)
Again it's difficult to say what is normal, since the amount of blood-loss varies from woman to woman and throughout life. You will know what is normal for you. If you pass large clots, soak the sheets at night, or blood gushes through clothing in the daytime and this is not usual for you, then seek help.

The commonest reasons for excessive bleeding are hormonal imbalance, IUDs, fibroids or polyps, endometriosis, obesity, certain rare blood diseases, stress and very occasionally cancer. You'll find some of these dealt with elsewhere. In this section I'll just look at heavy bleeding that has no apparent cause, often known as 'dysfunctional uterine bleeding'.

Dysfunctional uterine bleeding often accompanies cycles in which no egg is produced (anovulatory). It's most likely to occur during the early years of your periods and if you are over 35. Though you may bleed heavily, it's not usually especially painful. Serious causes are rare, especially in the first few years of menstruation, and the condition usually settles down by itself in time.

Heavy, irregular bleeding or bleeding that starts after you have completed the menopause could be a more serious sign, so you should always see your doctor.

Orthodox treatment
This consists of hormone treatment, the Pill, drugs that inhibit prostaglandin synthesis such as mefenamic acid (Ponstan), or drugs that increase the strength of the capiliary walls. The problem is that since these don't treat underlying causes your heavy periods will probably return once you stop taking the therapy.

D & C (dilatation and curettage), where the lining of the uterus is scraped out, or endometrial aspiration, where it is sucked out, used to be a common treatment for heavy periods. However these have been shown to have little long-term effect, though they may well be used for purposes of diagnosis. Sometimes, where periods are extremely heavy and don't respond to treatment, hysterectomy is performed. For details of this operation see pages 133-4.

Alternative therapies and self help
Having ruled out more serious problems, pay close attention to your diet. A lack of vitamin A has been suggested as one cause of heavy periods, and, if you favour nutritional methods, see a nutritionally oriented practitioner. Make sure, too, you get plenty of green leafy vegetables, wheatgerm, liver, parsley and other iron-rich foods to counteract the possible anaemia caused by excessive blood loss.

The stress measures outlined before will help you to relax — meditation and yoga can be especially useful. Both acupuncture and osteopathy have been used in the treatment of menorrhagia.

Herbal remedies that rebalance the hormones are used. David Hoffman in *The Holistic Herbal* (Findhorn) recommends an infusion of 1 part American Cranesbill, 1 part Beth Root, 1 part Periwinkle to be taken three times a day. For further advice consult a qualified herbalist.

Periods pains (dysmenorrhoea)
Periods pains can range from mild to severely disabling. How they affect you depends on your individual pain threshold and what else is going on in your life at the time. As always, stress can make them worse.

Doctors have divided period pains into two types: primary dysmenorrhoea which starts within a couple of years of beginning to menstruate, and secondary dys- menorrhoea which begins later in life. In primary dysmenorrhoea you experience a low cramp that may spread to your thighs and back, and you may also faint, feel sick or sweaty, or suffer constipation.

Secondary dysmenorrhoea tends to start with a general aching in your abdomen about a week to ten days before your period begins, and often goes hand in hand with other premenstrual symptoms. It may stop as soon as your periods starts or last all the way through it. The two types are considered to have different causes. Primary is thought to be a result of the uterus contracting, rather as it does when you are in labour, under the influence of prostaglandins. Secondary dysmenorrhoea has more wide ranging causes which may include pelvic inflammatory disease, endometriosis, fibroids, polyps or an infection. These are all dealt with elsewhere in this book.

Conventional treatment
For primary dysmenorrhoea, regular doses of aspirin, which act as a muscle relaxant and may improve blood flow to the uterus, anti-prostaglandin drugs such as mefenamic acid (Ponstan), or putting you on the Pill are all common. For secondary dysmenorrhoea you may be offered antibiotics, hormone treatment or surgery, depending on the cause.

Self help and alternative treatments

● Hold a covered hot water bottle against your abdomen.

● Take a warm bath or shower.

● Practice relaxation techniques.

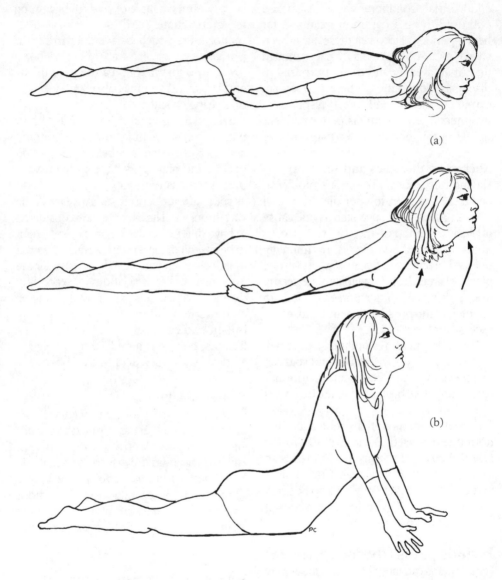

(a)

(b)

Figure 5: (a) The two steps of the cobra-exercise, to relieve menstrual cramps.
         (b) The bow exercise, to relieve muscle tension.

● Exercise, especially swimming, dance or yoga may all be beneficial. Lying with your legs up against a wall can help relieve that dragging feeling. Ask your yoga teacher to recommend suitable asanyas. The cobra (illustrated opposite) is especially useful, as is the bow.

● Visualization is useful when dealing with any sort of pain. Two exercises recommended by Vernon Coleman in *Natural Pain Control* (Century), could help:

1. Imagine your right hand is icy cold. When it feels numb place it over the painful area and let the numbness soak through.
2. Clasp your right hand as tightly as you can and imagine it is your uterus. Slowly relax it completely. As you do so, your uterus will relax and the pain should gradually ebb away.

It takes a little while to get the hang of using visualization techniques in this way, and you'll need to practise before trying to use them for pain relief.

● Direct massage of the uterus, done by pressing into your abdomen just above the pubic hairs and massaging gently, helps the uterus to relax. You may notice that this causes a large clot to be passed which then relieves pain.

● Herbal treatments include raspberry leaf tea, which you can buy from the health food store. It's an excellent tonic for the uterus. David Hoffmann, in *The Holistic Herbal*, recommends a mixture of 2 parts Black Haw Bark, 2 parts Cramp Bark, 1 part Pasque flower taken three times a day as an infusion.

● Some self-help homoeopathic remedies that may be useful are calc carb (if you have sore breasts), calc phos (if you have a headache), lycopodium (with depression), nat mur (if you are down and irritable) and pulsatilla (if you are weepy and have painful breasts). If none of these apply consult a homoeopath.

● Acupressure. Direct pressure on the Achilles tendon relieves tension and discomfort. (See illustration.)

● Shiatsu massage. Get a friend or your partner to press with the flat of the thumb on either side of the spinal column from your tail bone to your waist.

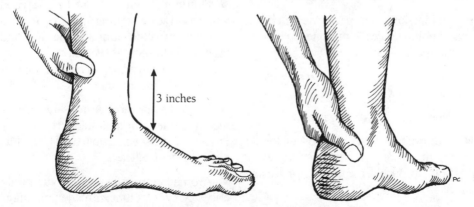

Figure 6: Position of acupressure point to relieve menstrual cramps.

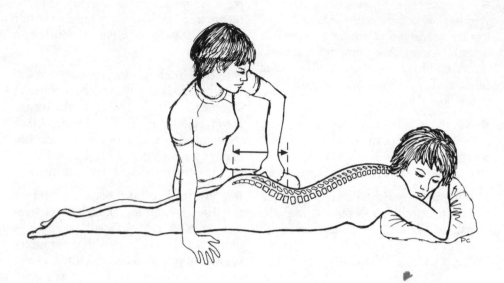

Figure 7: Shiatsu massage for menstrual pain relief.

● To relieve constipation, try squeezing half a lemon in some warm water and drink within half an hour of waking up.

● An infusion of ginger — one pinch to a cup of boiling water with honey to taste — during the period is useful.

● Osteopathy can help by freeing blood flow to the pelvis.

● Reflexology is also helpful.

● Acupuncture is especially useful for the treatment of any menstrual problems, possibly through its endorphin-releasing effect.

● TENS (Transcutaneous Electrical Nerve Stimulation) is extremely effective for period pains (see page 127).

● Nutritional remedies include a good wholefood diet, fasting, and perhaps a supplement of calcium, magnesium and vitamin D. However, as I've said before, trying to dose yourself with supplements is unwise, so consult a practitioner.

● The following biochemic tissue salts are recommended for painful periods: Mag Phos, Ferr Phos, Kali Phos, Calc Phos, Kali Mur, Nat Mur, Silica.

● Aromatherapy oils include: camomile, clary sage, cypress, juniper, marjoram, lemon, rosemary.

Fibroids

Fibroids affect about one in five of us over the age of 35. They are non-cancerous lumps that grow in the wall of the uterus. Very often if the fibroids are small they cause no trouble at all. But occasionally they can grow much larger — a large fibroid can weigh as much as 20 lbs! In this this case they may be responsible for heavy periods, bladder irritation, bleeding between periods and infertility. Fibroids are dependent on oestrogen and will shrink after the menopause.

If the fibroids are small and not causing you any bother they can usually safely be left alone. In fact you may not even know you have them except perhaps if a doctor comments that you have a 'bulky' uterus during an examination. Surgical removal is usually advised for very large fibroids or where you are experiencing a lot of heavy bleeding or pain. Usually just the fibroid will be removed (myomectomy), which means that you can still have children. But an exceptionally large fibroid may mean a hysterectomy. Is there anything you can do to avoid this?

The answer seems to be a qualified 'yes'. One medically qualified alternative practitioner told me, 'If the space occupied is big, the only thing to do is whip them out.

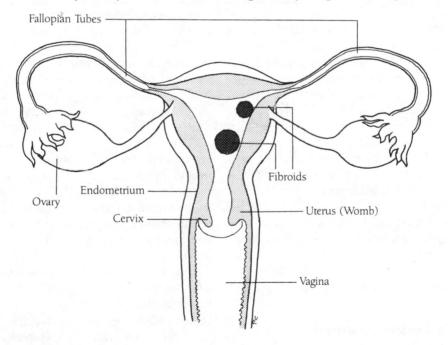

Figure 8: Common fibroid sites.

If the fibroid is small a sophisticated homoeopathic or herbal approach may even bring about reversal.' He emphasizes that there is no scientific proof of this, and that if such treatment is going to work it should have done so within about six months.

A psychotherapist I spoke to, who uses visualization techniques, also reported some striking results, 'The fibroid is often serving some purpose. For instance, one writer I saw found that the fibroid was to do with her creative blocks. The woman has to develop a different relationship with her condition, and not see the fibroid as something that shouldn't be there, but explore what sort of meaning it has.' She reported several cases where fibroids had shrunk after psychotherapy combined with visualization.

Of course such accounts are only anecdotal. But since we know that fibroids are oestrogen related, and since we also know that hormone imbalances can be brought on by stress, could it be that the reduction of stress brought about by psychotherapy is the explanation for the shrinkage of the fibroids?

Endometriosis

Endometriosis affects between one to five million women in this country, and is a major cause of heavy painful periods. It occurs when parts of the lining of the uterus (endometrium) attach themselves to other areas of the pelvis — often the ovaries, Fallopian tubes or the outside of the uterus. The patches of lining grow and bleed each cycle just as if they were still inside the womb, under the influence of the hormones controlling menstruation. The blood, which is not able to be disposed of in the usual way, forms scabs and scar tissue, which cause parts of the pelvic organs to stick together (adhesions). Apart from heavy painful periods, pain between periods, deep pain during intercourse, backache and infertility are signs of endometriosis.

Orthodox treatment and diagnosis

A laparoscopy which enables the doctor to look at your reproductive organs will show up small blood-filled cysts, or larger masses known as 'chocolate cysts.' Usually treatment consists of stopping hormonal action. Pregnancy can be a temporary respite because of high levels of circulating progesterone. If you want a baby the doctor may recommend you to get pregnant fairly soon, especially as you could eventually become infertile if the condition worsens.

Orthodox treatment consists of putting you on a high dose pill, or progesterone type hormones. A common treatment is by means of the drug danazol (Danol) which suppresses the function of the pituitary which controls the menstrual hormones, and in large enough doses can cause the lesions to shrink. The trouble is that the treatment is long winded, expensive and has a whole host of extremely unpleasant side effects including weight gain, acne, skin rashes, headaches, muscle cramps and hairiness. A new nasal contraceptive which is said to be suitable for treating endometriosis is at present being tried out. It is called Buserelin and works by preventing the pituitary from releasing luteinising hormone (LH) which is involved in ovulation. Buserelin stops both ovulation and menstruation. But side effects include hot flushes and a dry vagina — the typical menopausal symptoms thought to be caused by low oestrogen levels. What's more, the new treatment is unlikely to be available for a few years.

Surgical treatment consists of scraping off the areas affected by endometriosis and freeing any organs trapped by adhesions. If the endometriosis is not widespread and if you want a family this may be a worthwhile solution. As a last resort you may be offered hysterectomy and occasionally removal of your ovaries (oophorectomy). If your ovaries are removed, then you will experience a premature menopause.

Alternative treatment and self-help

The Endometriosis Society believes the key to the future lies in earlier diagnosis and the prevention of tissue damage, adhesions and infertility which cause so much physical pain and heartache. A leaflet put out by the Society makes the following point: 'Many women do not feel or realise that persistently painful periods, painful bowel movements or painful sexual intercourse are very good reasons for visiting their GPs. Women may be embarrassed, worry about wasting the doctor's time or simply disregard these symptoms in the mistaken belief that they are a normal part of being a woman.'

Alternative treatment is three pronged:

— restoration of health and well-being which has been undermined by months or years of pain and heavy blood loss

— soothing pain and alleviating symptoms
— restoring hormone balance.

In a sheet put out by the Endometriosis Society the following *alternative therapies* are recommended:

● Diet and vitamin therapy. Calcium and magnesium supplements (dolomite) in the week before your period can alleviate cramps. High doses of vitamin C with added bioflavonoids are said to compensate for high oestrogen levels and reduce blood flow. Supplements of A, B and E vitamins, plus zinc and selenium are also said to be helpful, as is the ever versatile evening primrose oil.

● Biochemic tissue salts

● Homoeopathy.

● Herbal medicine. Chaste Tree (*vitex agnus castus*) is perhaps the most useful treatment since it normalizes the action of the pituitary gland, and especially progesterone production. Teas such as Camomile, St John's Wort, Marigold, Lady's Mantle, Raspberry and Hops, Fennel and Yarrow are recommended. However, since endometriosis is potentially so serious you are advised to seek the help of a medically qualified herbalist and not to try and treat yourself.

● Yoga may be especially helpful through its relaxing effects, and because it can alter hormone production and restore the nervous system.

● Visualization. The following visualization exercise is suggested in the Endometriosis Society leaflet:

'We should think of ways in which we might consciously look after our needs more (as women we have usually been taught that our needs come second) so that we no longer need endometriosis to do that for us. We can consciously use our minds' resources to overcome the illness. We can start by breathing down 'into our stomachs' and relaxing each part of the body in turn from head to toe, and then visualize ourselves in a pleasant natural setting. From there, we can move on to visualize the weak, confused endometriosis cells (lost in the wrong place) and the strong purposeful army of white blood cells flooding in with increased blood flow, destroying the endometriosis cells and getting rid of them, soothing pain and tidying up scar tissue. We can visualize our internal organs, pink and healthy, freely mobile, and balanced hormones and see ourselves, healthy and full of energy, achieving the goals we want.'

You can do this for a quarter of an hour about three times a day.

● Nutritional methods — DLPA (Phenylalanine) is a new discovery from America which strengthens and protects the body's natural pain killers, endorphins. It's a mixture of two forms of the amino acid (Phenylalanine) and is said to be as powerful as morphine, while at the same time being non-addictive, and having no side effects. It also seems to help in cases of depression, which is a common feature of endometriosis, as a result of constant pain.

You can get it from health food stores, or Nature's Best Health Products Ltd, PO Box 1, 1 Lamberts Road, Tunbridge Wells, Kent. (1986 price 60 capsules £7.70).

● Acupuncture can ease pain and help normalize the menstrual cycle.

● Reflexology and aromatherapy may also be used.

Further information:
The Endometriosis Society, 65 Holmdene Avenue, Herne Hill, London SE24 9LD Tel: 01-737-4764.

Produces extremely useful fact sheets, send s.a.e. for details of prices and so on.

Premenstrual Syndrome

From being virtually unrecognized, premenstrual syndrome (PMS) — or premenstrual tension (PMT) as it is sometimes still called — has received a blast of publicity in both the popular and medical press. It's been estimated that nine out of ten of us may suffer PMS. But even though PMS is at last receiving serious recognition, confusion as to causes and treatments abounds.

The hormonal clue

What seems cast-iron is that those of us who suffer PMS react in some way to the hormonal changes of the menstrual cycle. But that isn't to say that PMS is *caused* by our hormones. We still don't know the exact relationship between hormones and PMS, nor how diet, pollution, stress, lifestyle and personality affect it.

Some experts claim that it's the rises and falls in hormone levels that create PMS. According to this view, oestrogen encourages water retention, while prolactin, released by the pituitary under stress is responsible for breast tenderness. Hormones affect neurotransmitters (chemical messengers) in the brain, especially serotonin which is responsible for feelings of serenity and tranquillity. It's argued that the fall in serotonin levels causes the feelings of anxiety, depression and so on.

Perhaps the most vociferous promoter of hormonal theories is endocrinologist Katharina Dalton, who believes PMS is caused by progesterone deficiency. However, Dr Dalton's views are controversial, even amongst orthodox medics. Endocrine changes can *result* from physical or mental stress rather than being caused by them, and some studies have shown that women with very low concentrations of progesterone do not suffer PMS.

Another theory suggested that prosta-glandins produced in the uterus were responsible for the typical cluster of symptoms. However it's recently been found that cyclical mental and physical symptoms can carry on after hysterectomy, neatly putting paid to that idea.

An intriguing theory outlined in 'Not all in the Mind', a pamphlet produced by the Women's Health Information Centre, suggests that at certain levels hormones act on the brain causing a higher level of arousal. Whether you experience this state as positive or negative depends on what else is happening in your life at the time. For instance if you are under a lot of stress, you will interpret the arousal as negative. If you are feeling loved, supported and cherished, the time before your period may bring feelings of well-being, increased energy and elation. This theory makes a lot of sense in view of the many contradictory emotions

women with PMS suffer.

The food connection

Diet seems to play a major role in PMS. Symptoms get worse if you skip meals, and food cravings, especially for sweet things, are common, as is increased appetite. Even orthodox doctors accept that there is a diet connection. In particular, shortages of vitamin B_6, magnesium, iron and zinc have been implicated. It's known that the Pill, too much coffee and tea, sugar and alcohol can deplete the body of essential nutrients. Coffee and smoking in particular may increase breast tenderness and swelling as well as affecting mood.

Professor Guy Abrahams, formerly Professor of Obstetrics and Gynaecology at the University of California believes PMS is caused by these three factors:

● diet

● hormone imbalances

● stress.

He divides sufferers into four types:

TYPE A: Anxiety, irritability, tension

TYPE B: Bloating, swelling, weight gain

TYPE C: Cravings for sweets and stodgy foods, followed by exhaustion, headache, fainting brought about by sudden rises and falls in blood sugar (hypoglycaemia).

TYPE D: Depression and confusion.

The Sussex based PMT Advisory Service recommends diets and menus specially tailored to the four different types. The only catch is that many of us don't fit that easily into any one of these categories.

Who gets PMS?

You're more likely to have PMS if:

☐ You are over 30.

☐ You have two or more children.

☐ Your mother was a PMS sufferer.

☐ You have recently experienced a hormone upheaval — for example having a baby, coming off the Pill, being sterilized, if you've been anorexic.

☐ You have had several pregnancies in quick succession.

Treatment

The line between orthodox treatment and alternative treatment is fast becoming blurred. Many of the PMS clinics mentioned below offer alternative treatments such as B_6 supplements and evening primrose oil, plus advice on relaxation and so on. Antidepressants and tranquillizers, formerly widely used by conventional doctors are out, after studies showed them to have no value over a placebo. It's probably helpful to think of treatment on a continuum for orthodox to alternative. If you have PMS it's probably a question of finding the right combination of treatment for you. The picture is made even more complicated by the fact that at least 50 per cent of women improve even when given a placebo.

Main lines of treatment are as follows:

Psychotherapy

A recent article in the doctors' newspaper *Pulse* says: 'Counselling, advice, psychotherapy and above all sympathetic under-

standing form the mainstay of management and may be the only treatment necessary'.

Diet

This is more controversial. PMS expert Michael Brush advises a good wholefood diet, free of additives. The PMT Advisory Service goes one step further, and will supply you with individually tailored diet sheets. The service doesn't come cheap, so it may be worth following the diet guidelines outlined in the box (page 60), before forking out large sums of money.

Vitamin B_6

A special mention should be made of vitamin B_6. Dr Michael Brush claims that 70 per cent of PMS sufferers can be helped by supplements of B_6 (pyridoxine). Dr Alan Stewart of the PMT Advisory Service recommends supplements of this and other B complex vitamins, plus magnesium supplements. However, Dr Katharina Dalton is outspoken in her claim that large supplements of B_6 can cause nervous system symptoms such as tingling or numbness, that disappear once the supplement is stopped. It's probably true to say that megadoses (over 200mg of B_6 *a day*) should only be carried out under the supervision of a nutritionally based practitioner. But smaller doses as outlined should be safe.

● Take 50mg tablets twice a day. You can increase the dose but don't go above 200mg a day unless you are under the supervision of a qualified practitioner.

● Begin the tablets three days before symptoms usually start and continue until the second or third day of your period, or until the symptoms normally stop. If your periods are irregular it is safe to take the tablets every day.

● Continue for three or four months then stop to see whether they have helped. If they have you can safely continue.

● If the method doesn't work, or if you experience side effects such as numbness or tingling, stop the treatment and consult your doctor or an alternative practitioner.

● If you get pregnant stop taking the supplement, as there is a suggestion that large amounts might cause birth defects.

Evening primrose oil
Trials at St Thomas's Hospital have long suggested that over 60 per cent of women with PMS can be helped by taking evening primrose oil. It's especially useful if you suffer breast discomfort, eczema, irritability, depression or if you are diabetic. You shouldn't take it if you suffer from epilepsy.

Evening primrose oil is thought to work by means of a rare essential fatty acid (gammalinoleic acid or GLA for short) that converts into prostaglandin E in the body. A diet too rich in animal fats, processed oils and alcohol, as well as certain viruses, cancer and exposure to radiation all affect the body's ability to form GLA, and may explain why many women are short of it.

Side effects are uncommon, but some women experience diarrhoea or stomach upsets, and a few are allergic to the gelatine which is used in the capsule, in which case you can get drops.

Take two 500mg capsules twice a day after food, starting three days before symptoms usually start. You may need more or less, depending on how you respond, and advice on this can be found in *The Premenstrual Syndrome — The Curse that Can be Cured*, by

Dr Caroline Shreeve (Thorsons), Evening primrose oil is made more effective if you take it with a vitamin and mineral supplement such as Efavite, which contains vitamin B_6, vitamin C and zinc.

Does it work?
These are some of the comments made in a *Here's Health* study of the effectiveness of evening primrose oil:
'Stomach cramps and bloated stomach disappeared.'
'Premenstrual symptoms greatly reduced in first month and almost disappeared in second.'
'Headache and other symptoms worse.'
'Dramatic effect. No monthly "row" with husband.'
'Period pain reduced from severe to absent. Will buy if I can afford.'

Further information:
Naudicelle Capsules, Bio Oil Research Ltd, The Hawthorns, 64 Welsh Row, Nantwich, Cheshire CW5 5VE.

Not available on prescription, but if your doctor recommends use you can get exemption from VAT by sending his signature on your order.

Other supplements
Vitamin E can help some women (take 150-600 IU a day). Magnesium supplements are also helpful for some women, though unfortunately you can only get a very crude form of this on the NHS, so consult a reliable alternative practitioner or write to the PMT Advisory Service for details. Dr Alan Stewart of the PMT Advisory Service advises a multivitamin-mineral preparation called Optivite.

What you eat

Observe the following good food rules:

● Eat whole grains, nuts and seeds. Almonds, coconut, sesame and sunflower seeds provide potassium which may be depleted if you have PMS.

● Avoid tea, coffee, cocoa, coke-type drinks and alcohol. Substitute spring water and herb teas.

● Eat small, frequent meals to dispel sugar cravings and keep up blood sugar levels.

● Include plenty of raw foods in what you eat.

● Limit dairy foods as they may interfere with magnesium absorption. Good sources of magnesium include green leafy vegetables and lentils.

● Cut out junk foods, sweets, cakes and pastries: they can cause water retention and prevent the body absorbing essential minerals.

● Cut salt intake, if bloating is a problem.

Hormone treatments

These may include the Pill — though many doctors think that this actually aggravates symptoms, and artificial and natural hormones of the progesterone family such as dydrogesterone (Duphaston) and norethisterone (Primolut N). However, side effects are off-putting, including breast tenderness, headaches, varicose veins, piles, and vaginal infections. Dr Katharina Dalton argues that only pure progesterone in the form of suppositories or injections should be used. But many doctors disagree, and progesterone can cause unwelcome side effects.

Danazol, which is described in the section on endometriosis, may also be prescribed, though for many women the side effects are worse than the PMS.

Oestradiol implants

The newest and most controversial treatment aims to suppress ovulation in an attempt to control hormonal fluctuations. It involves placing an implant of oestradiol, a type of oestrogen, under the skin of your stomach. Mr John Studd of Kings College Hospital believes it's the *only* treatment for severe PMS. Many orthodox doctors violently disagree. It can cause period irregularities, and other problems which may be very hard to deal with once the implant is there. Mr Studd is unrepentant — he claims the side effects of breast pain, nausea, weight gain and headache are usually mild and temporary! You pays your money and you takes your choice.

Non-hormone drug therapies

These include anti prostaglandins such as mefenamic acid (Ponştan) and bromocriptine, which dampens down prolactin production. However, bromocriptine can cause vomiting and some doctors believe it is dangerous. The use of diuretics to get rid of swelling is also recommended by some doctors though others argue that this doesn't really treat the root cause of PMS and only deals with a symptom. What's more diuretics can leach the body of potassium.

Herbal remedies

There are numerous herbal treatments for PMS. Scullcap and valerian in tablet form can ease tension. Dandelion, though bitter, can help with fluid retention. Potters PMT tablets, available from the health food shop or the address on page 145, contain vervain, gentian, motherwort, meadow anemone, bearberry and valerian. But perhaps the treatment of choice again is *vitex agnus castus* (Chase tree), a progesterone-like herb that helps improve pituitary function and hormone levels. Go to a qualified herbal practitioner for all but the simplest treatments.

Homoeopathic treatment

This is often very successful. The following self-help remedies have been suggested: calc carb (with tender breasts), graphites (with weight gain), lycopodium (with depression), nat mur (with irritability), nux vom (if you are argumentative), pulsatilla (if you are weepy), sepia (if you suffer mood swings). You are advised to consult a qualified homoeopath, who will look at you as a whole and try to find the best remedy for you as a person.

Acupuncture and acupressure

Both see PMS as a result of imbalance or blockage of vital energy or chi, and there are many excellent results reported from using them.

Osteopathy, reflexology, aromatherapy can all help too.

Self help

Smoking
A recent study reported in the *British Medical Journal* reports that smoking interferes with blood flow, and increases the secretion of stress hormones. Evening primrose oil was shown to improve blood flow in smokers. Better still — try and give up altogether!

Stress
Stress can deplete magnesium in the body, so follow the stress relieving tips outlined earlier. Yoga, meditation, T'ai chi, dance are just some of the therapies that may be useful.

A menstrual diary
Keep a diary for three to four months, either on the lines of the one illustrated, or a written record, if you find that easier. Note mood changes and physical symptoms. Record feelings of well-being and energy, as well as more negative feelings. It's all too easy to record a bout of irritability coming before a period, but dismiss such a mood as unimportant afterwards. What you're aiming for is an *awareness* of mood fluctuations over the whole of your cycle.

Managing your moods
Once you've got a picture of your mood changes, you can start to deal with them. PMS may alert you to issues in your life that need attention. The feelings of frustration, anger, hopelessness and so on many of us feel premenstrually aren't entirely negative. They can be valuable pointers to areas of your life that need tackling.

Of course there may be some problems you can't do anything about. You may be struggling to manage on too little money, feeling isolated or overwhelmed by the demands of young children for example. But that doesn't mean these problems don't matter. Women often feel it's wrong, or 'unfeminine' to be angry. Accepting your right to be angry or depressed may help you feel less stressed. Seeing that a problem that you thought just affected you is more widespread may prompt you to join a group working for wider change.

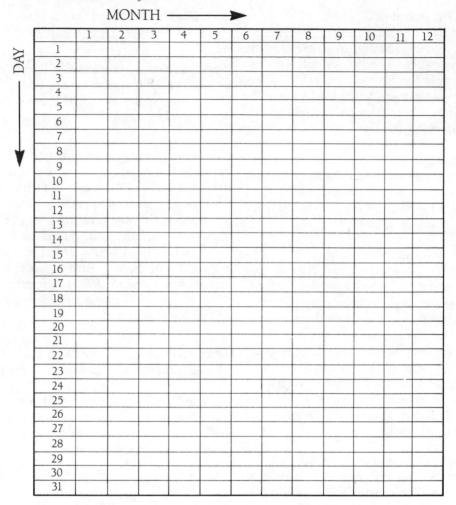

DAY \ MONTH	1	2	3	4	5	6	7	8	9	10	11	12
1												
2												
3												
4												
5												
6												
7												
8												
9												
10												
11												
12												
13												
14												
15												
16												
17												
18												
19												
20												
21												
22												
23												
24												
25												
26												
27												
28												
29												
30												
31												

During which month did you start recording your symptoms?...................................

Indicate each day of your menstruation with an 'M' in the appropriate square.

Indicate each day on which you experience symptoms by using the relevant letters from this key —

D — Depression   T — Tension, Irritability or Anxiety
P — Pain (backache or headache)   BT — Breast Tenderness
F — Fatigue   B — Bloated Feeling

Figure 9: Example of a menstrual diary.

On a more personal level, dealing with your emotions might include psychotherapy to help you identify and deal with problems that upset you premenstrually, counselling or assertiveness training to help you cope with anger more constructively.

Try to make life easy for yourself in the run up to your period. Save heavy jobs around the house, difficult meetings at work, awkward discussions until after your period if you can. Meditation, a warm bath, a walk, talking to a friend, painting, sex (with a partner or by masturbation) can all help release tension and help you relax.

Support and help
Enlist the help of friends and family at this time. Join a PMS support group, or seek out a special PMS clinic or alternative practitioner.

Some outside sources of help include:
NHS PMS Clinics
(Note: you may have to be referred by your G.P. to one of these.)
St George's Hospital, London SW17
Elizabeth Garrett Anderson Hospital, London NW1 (specializes in women)
Whitely Wood Clinic, Sheffield S10
Leeds General Infirmary, Leeds 1

Private Services
Marie Stopes Clinic, London WC1 (offers naturopathic and osteopathic treatments)
PMS Advisory Service, PO Box 268, Hove, E. Sussex BN3 1RW (counselling, personal diet profiles etc)

Headaches and Migraine
Migraine affects one in five of us and is more common in women than men. If you suffer headaches or migraine you are most likely to have them in the week leading up to your period. The highest incidence of headaches and migraine is found in those on the Pill. The Migraine Trust list a number of triggers for an attack which include:

● Alcohol.

● Fried or fatty food, pork, pickled herring, Marmite.

● Skipping meals.

● Certain types of food commonly chocolate, cheese and dairy products, citrus fruits, vegetables, tea and coffee, meat, sea food.

That's not to say that food is the sole reason for all migraine attacks, some people simply seem to be born with a tendency to it.

Tension headaches are often brought on by physical or mental stress, for example driving a car with your head held in the same position for a long time.

Research is currently being carried out at St Thomas's Hospital, London to see whether there is a hormone connection between certain types of headache and migraine. In the meantime the following *self help and alternative* methods may help.

● Keep a diary so that you can see if there is a pattern to the headaches.

● Don't skip meals, especially breakfast.

● Try to get a 'proper' meal at lunchtime.

● Eat regularly, if you're going out in the evening, try to have something to eat before you go.

● If you develop an attack try to eat something as lack of food makes it worse.

● Acupuncture or acupressure.

● Reflexology.

● Therapeutic touch (laying on of hands).

● Herbal medicine — the ancient herbal remedy Feverfew has recently received the thumbs up from conventional medicine. You can either eat Feverfew in a sandwich or make it into a tea, or get it in tablet form from the health shop. The Migraine Trust produce a leaflet on Feverfew.

● Homoeopathic dosages of Feverfew are now available, and there are a number of other homoeopathic remedies.

● Biochemic tissue salts.

● Yoga has a number of useful postures.

● Meditation and relaxation.

Do you suffer from PMS?

Over 150 symptoms have been listed by PMS sufferers. Below are the most frequently mentioned ones. How many of them apply to you?

☐ Feelings of depression, sadness, pessimism.
☐ Tiredness, lethargy, feelings of being 'under the weather'.
☐ Tension, irritability, anxiety.
☐ Increased or decreased appetite.
☐ Craving for sweet or salty foods.
☐ Thirst.
☐ Lack of concentration, difficulties in decision-making.
☐ Weepiness
☐ Moodswings.
☐ Feeling extra sexy or losing interest in sex.
☐ Inability to sleep or wanting to sleep all the time.
☐ Aggressive outbursts, impulsive behaviour.
☐ Increased energy.
☐ Loss of confidence and self-esteem, wanting to stay indoors all the time.
☐ Guilt feelings, putting yourself down.

☐ Loss of interest in yourself.
☐ Apathy.
☐ Headache or migraine.
☐ Breast swelling and tenderness.
☐ Bloating or feeling of bloatedness.
☐ Swollen fingers and toes.
☐ Acne, rashes, itching.
☐ Constipation, nausea, diarrhoea.
☐ Poor coordination, clumsiness, becoming 'accident-prone'.
☐ Muscle weakness, backache, muscle pain.
☐ Dizziness.
☐ Weight gain.
☐ Increased sweatiness.
☐ Blurred vision, sore eyes.
☐ Passing an increased or decreased amount of urine.
☐ Pain low in the abdomen.
☐ Increased vaginal discharge.
☐ Decreased efficiency.

Based on *The Premenstrual Syndrome*, by Maurice Katz, (Update Postgraduate Centre Series, Update Publications, 1984).

Dealing with anger

It can be good sometimes to let off steam, but often, especially if you have PMS, anger can appear to be controlling you. Learning how to manage your anger can give you greater control over a situation.

STEP ONE: Identify situations that get you angry and work out exactly what it is that annoys you, and how you normally deal with it.

STEP TWO: Involves what an anger control expert — yes, there really is such a thing — calls 'changing your inner dialogue'. In other words you talk yourself through difficult confrontations.

Ready. . .

Say to yourself: 'I know that this is going to get me cross, but I know how to deal with it'. 'I can use my energy to manage this situation'. 'Keep my sense of humour'. It may feel a little artificial at first, but you'll soon get used to it, and think of statements of your own.

. . . Steady . . .

As you go into the confrontation remind yourself:
'I am going to stay calm'. 'There's no point in building a mountain out of a molehill. I can cope'.

. . . Go!

While you're doing this continue to monitor how you feel:
'I can feel my muscles getting tense. Relax'. 'Take it step by step'.

STEP THREE: Once the fray is over, think positive about the incident:
'It's all over now, I can forget about it'. 'I didn't do too badly that time. Next time I'll do even better'. Don't blame yourself if you did lose your cool. Breathe deeply and resolve to try again next time. If you did manage to cope with the situation, congratulate yourself — you deserve it!

Vaginal Infections

The vagina is self-cleansing and all of us secrete mucus made up of cells from the vagina and cervix. At certain times in our lives — for instance in our teens, during pregnancy, at certain times during the menstrual cycle, during sexual arousal and when you are on the Pill, the discharge can increase. A normal vaginal discharge is clear and sticky, whitish-yellow, or white and creamy, depending on the stage of your menstrual cycle. A daily wash of your genital area is sufficient to keep clean under most normal conditions, and there's no need to wash inside your vagina itself. However, if the discharge becomes different in colour or texture, and especially if the amount is more than usual or smelly you could have an infection. This section gives a run-down of the causes of vaginal discharge, non-infectious and infectious varieties, and the orthodox and alternative treatments.

Once the cause of the discharge is removed, the symptoms will disappear of their own accord (see 'Preventing vaginal infections' — page 70).

Non-infectious causes of vaginal discharge

● When just starting your periods

● Various different times during your menstrual cycle

● When you are sexually active

● During pregnancy

● During the menopause

● A forgotten tampon or other foreign body in the vagina

● Chemicals such as bubble baths, soap or douches

● Drug-related discharge e.g. if you are on the Pill, have been taking antibiotics or use contraceptive pessaries or gel

● Certain gynaecological problems such as cervical erosion

● Infectious causes of vaginal discharge

● Thrush

● Trichomonas (Trich)

● Bacterial infection (anaerobic vaginosis e.g. gardnerella)

● Chlamydia

● Herpes

● Gonorrhoea

Thrush (Monilia)

Thrush is caused by a fungal organism (candida albicans) that normally lives in places such as the vagina, back passage and under the fingernails, without causing any trouble. The fungus thrives in a sugary atmosphere, so that if the normally slightly acid environment of the vagina is disturbed in any way, it goes out of control. Times when this may occur are if you have a high intake of sugar in your diet, if you have diabetes, during pregnancy and during the second half of your menstrual cycle, if you are on a high-dose Pill. Some men's semen appears to be more alkaline than others, which may spark off an attack, especially if you have a new partner. A man with thrush can transmit it to you even if he has no symptoms himself. If you are run-down or under stress, an attack may be triggered off if you are susceptible. A course of antibiotics, by killing off the bacteria that normally keep candida in balance, often creates just the right conditions for thrush to grow.

Symptoms are a white cheesy discharge that smells yeasty. You may feel burning or pain on passing water. The discharge is usually sore and may be unbearably itchy, and you may have a rash that spreads to your inner thighs.

Orthodox diagnosis and treatment

The doctor will examine you — this may be sufficient to diagnose thrush. He may also want to take a swab to be analysed in the lab to rule out any other infections, and may also carry out a simple pH (acid-alkaline) test, using colour-sensitive paper to confirm whether the discharge is acid or alkaline. Treatment is with pessaries, cream and/or tablets (Canesten and Nystan being the most commonly used), and sometimes a special jelly to correct acid balance in the vagina. Occasionally where itchiness is extremely severe you may be given gentian violet. This is extremely soothing but beware — it's horribly messy!

Unfortunately, thrush has a nasty habit of coming back, unless you tackle the root causes, such as diet, stress or an unhealthy lifestyle. Women who suffer from recurrent thrush often feel thoroughly miserable and 'unclean'. Recurrent thrush continues to defy orthodox treatment, and the best your doctor will be able to do in many cases is to suggest long-term nystatin treatment. Many of us dislike the thought of being on medication virtually indefinitely, so what else can you do?

Self-help and alternative therapies

The answer is a combination of self-help and alternative treatment. The connection between recurrent thrush and stress, plus other facets of lifestyle, is crucial from the alternative viewpoint. Following the preventive tips outlined here will help cut your chances of developing an attack. At the first signs of a thrush attack:

● Bathe the vagina in a solution of one tablespoon of bicarbonate of soda to a pint of warm water. You can use a disposable douche to do this (empty out the contents first).

● Add salt to your bath — enough to make the water taste slightly salty.

● Take a vinegar bath — one part vinegar to three parts warm water — twice a day for a day or so to help rebalance the vaginal environment. Alternatively soak a tampon in the same quantities of solution and insert into your vagina. Never use neat vinegar as it will sting.

● Apply natural unsweetened live yogurt, using a tampon, applicator, plastic syringe or speculum. This is a slow but sure method — it takes some 10-15 days. Note though that some doctors in the USA have warned against this practice on the grounds that it can cause pregnancy complications. In any case you should never put anything in your vagina if you think you might be pregnant.

● Herbal remedies include compresses of golden seal, comfrey, crab apples, bay bark, myrrh, or thuja ointment from the health food store or a herbal supplier. Unless you are familiar with herbs and their uses consult a qualified herbalist, as all these remedies are expensive.

● Some practitioners recommend inserting a clove of garlic wrapped in muslin into your vagina. However some women have complained that this stings. Try it — but if it's too uncomfortable don't continue.

● Avoid sex with penetration until the thrush has cleared up.

Diet

A sugary diet, as I've already said, can predispose to thrush. Eat a good wholefood diet, and cut out alcohol and any foods containing mould or fungus such as Stilton cheese, mushrooms and so on. On a naturopathic regime you'll be advised to stay off fruit because of its high sugar content, and to take supplement of lactobacillus acidophilus — a bacteria which is killed by antibiotics. Vitamin B and C supplements may also be advised. Some experts recommend eating live yogurt, as well as applying it directly.

Homoeopathy

Homoeopathy has many useful remedies for vaginal discharge. A pilot study carried out in 1984 in orthodox clinics showed that a combination of two homoeopathic remedies, Borax and Candida, was significantly more effective than a placebo in treating certain women with thrush. It's not advised that you try to treat yourself with these, however, since they might not be indicated in your case.

The yeast connection

Some clinical ecologists (see page 141) go one step further and blame candida albicans (the organism involved in thrush) for being behind a whole host of other, seemingly unconnected ailments. These include diseases as apparently diverse as AIDS, Multiple Sclerosis, migraine, schizophrenia, PMS and arthritis. An article in the American Journal *Healthsharing*, Summer 1985 states: 'It's estimated that 30 per cent of the population is susceptible to severe candida infections. Women are affected more often than men.' The article blames modern lifestyle: antibiotics, the Pill, diet, chemicals at work and stress-related hormone imbalances for the epidemic of yeast related diseases.

According to this view such factors weaken the immune system, laying the body open for candida invasion. The way it affects you will depend on a number of factors including genetic susceptibility.

Advice consists of putting you on a diet low in sugary and starchy foods, as well as dried herbs and teas, pickled and smoked foods. Some practitioners also advise a bacterial product called Probion, developed in Scandinavia, to rebalance the flora in the gut and increase resistance to infection. Further details from The International Institute of Symbiotic Studies (see clinical ecology page 141).

It has to be said that this approach is highly controversial and most orthodox doctors would dismiss it entirely. As always,

in the absence of controlled trials, it's difficult to be certain. But if you do suffer from recurrent thrush for which no other treatment seems to work, it may well be worth consulting a clinical ecologist or other allergy specialist.

Trichomas vaginalis, TV or trich

Trich is caused by a one-celled organism, which like candida, is often already present in the vagina, anus, cervix, urethra or bladder, where it normally doesn't present problems. The discharge is frothy, yellowish-green with an unpleasant smell. You will be red and sore, and have a burning sensation when you pass water. Your cervix may be inflamed 'like a strawberry'. Trich is usually sexually transmitted, but you can catch it from other sources since it lives for several hours at room temperature in a moist atmosphere. For instance you could catch it from a wet swimsuit, toilet seat, towel or flannel that has been used by someone with trich.

The infection often goes with other sexually transmitted infections such as gonorrhoea. There's a high chance that your sex partner will be infected too, so both of you should be treated even if he or she has no apparent symptoms.

It may be worse immediately after or before your period because of the altered pH level in your vagina at this time. Like thrush, trich is more likely to take hold if you are already run down. If not treated properly it can ascend the Fallopian tubes causing pelvic inflammatory disease.

Bacterial vaginal infections (non-specific vaginitis)

Non-specific vaginitis is an umbrella term

used by doctors to describe a variety of bacterial infections. The commonest sort is perhaps gardnerella (corynebacterium vaginalis). Symptoms are a thin, watery, fishy-smelling discharge. The smell often gets worse mid-cycle or after sex. Your partner may be infected too but have no symptoms.

Orthodox treatment
Flagyl (metronidazole), a very powerful antibiotic, is the first line of treatment for both these infections. Alternatively for non-specific vaginitis other antibiotics are sometimes used, though these may be less effective and lead on to thrush. Flagyl is an extremely powerful drug, and it's important that you shouldn't take it during the first three months of pregnancy. It can have side-effects such as nausea, stomach upsets, headaches, and can also affect your white blood cell production. For this reason your doctor may want to take blood tests to see how you are responding to the drug. Flagyl also reacts with alcohol so you should cut out drinking.

Chlamydia
This is a fairly recently discovered virus-like bacteria. Younger women and those on the Pill are especially at risk. If left untreated it can lead to pelvic inflammatory disease (PID), a major cause of infertility.

Symptoms include a raised temperature, pain on opening your bowels and a pus or blood-stained discharge. Your cervix is inflamed, and there may be deep pelvic pain. If chlamydia is passed on to your unborn baby it can cause sticky eye after birth, breathing difficulties, and very occasionally even blindness.

The main problem with chlamydia is that it is often symptomless. If you have any reason to suspect that your partner may have an infection it's worth going for a test to your nearest STD clinic. Treatment is with powerful antibiotics such as Flagyl, tetracycline or erythromycin. Tetracycline shouldn't be used if you are pregnant as it can stain your baby's teeth yellow.

Gonorrhoea and syphilis
The two traditional venereal diseases (VD), though nowadays they come under the same umbrella as chlamydia, trichomonas and herpes: they are all STD's. Of the two, gonorrhoea is the most common and may be especially difficult to treat because it is often symptomless in women. If left untreated it's a major cause of blocked tubes leading on to sterility. It often goes hand in hand with chlamydia, and if you have one you should always be tested for the other, since treating the gonorrhoea alone may just mask the chlamydia with the subsequent risk of pelvic inflammatory disease developing. Where symptoms do appear they develop within five to seven days of sexual contact. You'll have an offensive yellow discharge, pain when you pass urine and frequency of urination.

Syphilis is rarer and even harder to detect. It has an incubation period of between two weeks and a month, and sometimes even longer. It's much commoner in men than women. If left untreated it can eventually lead on to diseases of the heart and nervous system. Symptoms start with a small painless sore that, left untreated, heals within six to ten weeks. You may get swollen glands in the groin, or other lymph glands. Treatment is with large doses of antibiotics, and if carried out at this early stage it is usually 100 per cent successful.

Preventing vaginal infections

If you practise self-examination as described in part one you may be able to spot an incipient infection before it gets chance to take hold, so you can immediately put a preventive plan into action.

● Pay attention to diet. In particular cut down sugary foods. A drink of a teaspoon of honey and vinegar in hot water will help maintain the vagina's normally slightly acid environment.

● Get plenty of rest and sleep.

● If you are run down or under stress, follow the stress management strategies outlined elsewhere. Meditation, yoga, T'ai chi or any of the mind-body therapies may be helpful.

● Avoid using flannels or sponges to wash the genital area as these can harbour germs.

● Always wipe from front to back after opening your bowels to prevent contamination of the vagina with bacteria from the anus.

● Avoid vaginal deodorant sprays, talc, scented soap and bubble or antiseptic bath solutions.

● Go for cotton underwear.

● Avoid tight jeans and knickers. Expose the area to air and sunlight if you get the opportunity!

● Take your swim things off immediately you get out of the water and allow them to dry.

● Keep your nails short and your hands clean.

● A cupful of vinegar in the bath water occasionally will help maintain the acid balance of your vagina.

● Make sure your partner keeps his penis and beneath the foreskin clean.

● Avoid coloured toilet rolls.

● Practise pelvic floor exercises as described in part one to increase circulation to the area.

● For relief of itching apply a compress of yogurt or cottage cheese several times a day. Alternatively bathe your genitals in a sage or chickweed infusion. For further details of herbal douches and compresses for vaginal infections see *The Holistic Herbal*, by David Hoffman, (Findhorn).

Alternative medicine and self-help

No lay practitioner is allowed by law to treat sexually transmitted diseases. However, there are plenty of things you can do to improve your resistance so that your body can fight off these infections more effectively. What's more, alternative treatments can provide a useful back-up to conventional treatment. An orthodox doctor who is also qualified in alternative therapies can of course treat you. Homoeopathy in particular has some useful remedies. A herbalist may advise douches and compresses, for instance of golden-seal, myrrh, comfrey to mention a few. Aromatherapy oils can be useful either taken by mouth or in a hip-bath, and can help increase the effectiveness of antibiotics. But all these are probably best used as an adjunct to conventional treatment rather than a first line.

Herpes

So far I've looked at bacterial infections. More difficult to treat are virus infections. The main one being herpes, or herpes simplex to give it its full name.

Genital herpes, or herpes 2, is a form of the virus herpes that causes cold sores around the mouth, and is now the second most common sexually transmitted disease, especially in women. So far there is no permanent cure, though there are many ways you can help keep herpes at bay or stem an attack should you develop one.

On the whole herpes is more a nuisance than dangerous, except that there is an as yet unproven suggestion that cervical cancer may be more common if you have herpes. Herpes can also be passed on to your unborn baby if you are pregnant. If this happens it can be very serious or even fatal to your baby. If you have open sores at the time of birth, you'll be advised to have a caesarean.

Herpes is often picked up through sexual contact, though not always. It may be transferred from mouth to genitals during oral sex, via the fingers or even on damp towels or flannels. The point to bear in mind is that you must have had some sort of contact with an open herpes sore. At this stage you will develop a first infection between two and twenty days after exposure. The commonest time is about a week after contact. The first attack of herpes is usually worst. The first sign is a tingling or burning sensation, followed by fluid-filled sores which burst to form ulcers, which then scab over and heal. You may develop swollen tender glands in your groin, a temperature, headache and general fluey feeling. The infection may last up to three weeks. Subsequent infections aren't usually so severe or long lasting. But once you have developed the sores the virus remains in your body where it can be re-activated, often if you are run down or under stress. Other triggers include having another illness which produces a high temperature, exposure to ultraviolet light e.g. when you sunbathe, menstruation or injury.

You are contagious from the time you feel the first signs until the sores have healed over completely.

Orthodox treatment

See your doctor as soon as the first symptoms appear so that he can take a swab. This is important to rule out the possibility of other STDs and confirm the diagnosis. If you do have herpes you'll be referred to a specialist STD clinic.

Orthodox treatment is limited at the

moment. It consists of anaesthetic gels or ointment to relieve pain, plus pain-killers such as aspirin or something stronger to be taken by mouth. You'll usually be given an anaesthetic jelly such as Xylocaine to smooth on before passing urine, to reduce burning and stinging. You may also be given antibiotics to prevent or treat any secondary bacterial infection you may have picked up. There are also a number of anti-viral drugs now available. The main trouble with these in the past has been that not only did they kill the virus but the cell along with it, so causing a number of unpleasant side-effects. The most promising new development is a drug called acyclovir (Zovirax) which seems according to the doctor's journal *The Practitioner* to be 'remarkably free of side-effects'. It seems to be effective in cutting short the length of the attack as well as the time taken for the sores to heal.

There are also reports of a new vaccine, not yet available on the NHS which may help prevent recurrent attacks.

But acyclovir can't prevent future attacks. It's only fair to say that many people experience just one episode of herpes and that's it. But some will go on to develop further attacks especially when run down or under stress.

So what does alternative medicine have to offer?

Self-help and alternative therapies
The alternative approach focuses on diet. Two amino acids arginine and lysine have been found to play a big part in preventing or encouraging attacks of herpes. A diet high in lysine found in foods such as fresh fish, chicken, cheese, lima beans, cottage cheese, beansprouts, prawns, has been found to inhibit attacks. A diet high in arginine found

in various types of nuts, sesame seeds, cocoa, brown rice, wholemeal bread, raisins and sunflower seeds, has been found to promote an outbreak. It's important to grasp that these foods don't cause herpes, but they may predispose you to an attack if you already have the virus in a dormant form.

Some naturopaths claim complete remission of the disease, but you have to follow treatment to the letter for it to be effective. Extra A, B, C and E vitamins may help prevent attacks.

The immune system
Your immune system is the other mainstay of any alternative approach to herpes. As North and Crittenden say in *Stop Herpes Now!* (Thorsons): 'A healthy immune system can keep the virus quietly under control . . . help your body resist infection from herpes — use good nutrition, exercise and conscious stress-reduction techniques to keep your immune system in top condition.'

Alternative techniques such as meditation, which can sometimes have a direct effect on the immune system, hypnosis, yoga, visualization techniques and relaxation can all help. Other therapies which have helped some people include homoeopathy, acupuncture and herbalism. Herbal treatments include an infusion of cloves, peppermint oil and clove oil, applied by a compress.

Self-help
● A warm bath or a hip-bath with salt added to relieve discomfort.

● Apply ice packs to the affected area.

● Wear cotton underwear.

● Keep the sores clean and dry. Wash with soap and water.

● Cold tea-bags can reduce inflammation.

● Pay attention to diet. Eat foods high in lysine and low in arginine.

High lysine foods: fish, chicken, beef, milk, lamb, pork, lima beans, cottage cheese, mung bean-sprouts, shrimps, prawns, soya beans, egg.

High arginine foods: hazelnuts, brazil nuts, peanuts, walnuts, almonds, cocoa, peanut butter, sesame seeds, cashew nuts, carob powder, coconut, pistachio nuts, buckwheat flour, chick peas, brown rice, pecan nuts, wholemeal bread, cooked oatmeal, raisins, sunflower seeds.

To prevent attacks

● Work out what triggers off an attack. Keeping a diary will help.

● Eat a diet high in raw foods and low in fat and sugar. Continue to eat high lysine foods or take lysine tablets available from the health food store.

● Avoid or deal with unnecessary stress.

● See a nutritionally qualified practitioner and find out if mineral supplements would benefit you.

● Visit a holistic G.P. or naturopath to find out about dietary changes you could make.

● See a medically qualified homoeopath. There are a number of homoeopathic remedies which may help.

To avoid herpes

● Don't touch cold sores around the mouth or genitals of a partner or friend.

● Don't share flannels, sponges, towels, lipstick or other intimate items with anyone else.

● If you have a new partner find out whether he or she has ever had herpes.

● Use barrier methods of contraception for safety.

● Don't have sex with penetration or masturbation when open sores are present.

● Pay attention to diet, exercise and stress management.

You and your partner
If you've had herpes in the past you may feel depressed and anxious, and as though you have no right to have sex. It's only fair to warn a new partner if you have had herpes. Open honest discussion of the risks of infection and how you can deal with the problem together will go a long way towards helping you deal with it. A Herpes Association pamphlet *Herpes simplex and you* stresses, 'Herpes is not you. You just have a rash which occasionally gets in the way. When you can handle the contagion problem, the emotional concerns will diminish.' Of course you can't entirely rule out the possibility of infecting your partner, but with sensible measures of the sort outlined above, you can reduce the risks to the minimum. Even if intercourse, masturbation or oral sex is out, there are

plenty of other ways you can enjoy each other sexually. Now is your chance to be creative, and find out new ways to please each other.

Genital warts

These are caused by a virus which is usually passed on sexually. They don't hurt, but they may itch or bleed. Vigorous sex or wearing tight fitting jeans can irritate them, and they thrive in a warm moist atmosphere. Genital warts (human papillomavirus or HPV) is a growing problem. Until recently they were considered only a minor nuisance, however recent studies have suggested a strong connection between HPV virus and the subsequent development of cancer of the cervix.

As with herpes there's no way of preventing recurrence. Conventional treatment consists of burning them off or the use of a caustic resin called podophyllum.

If you've had genital warts, you should make sure you go for regular smear-tests so that any early signs of cervical cancer can be treated at an early stage.

Alternative treatments

There's little information available on alternative treatments. However thuja ointment or tincture can be used, either by a herbalist or in homoeopathic doses. Mandrake root is also suggested. Acupuncture and homoeopathy can both help tone up the system so your body can throw off the infection more readily.

Other vaginal problems

Cervical erosion

When cells from inside the cervix (neck of the womb) grow on the outside, a red shiny area develops that may produce increased mucus. Sometimes the erosion may become infected.

Erosion occurs because of an excess of oestrogen. That means you are more likely to develop one if you are pregnant, on the Pill or at other times of hormonal upset, for instance if you are under stress.

Occasionally an erosion may bleed after sex, but it's usually painless, and you may not even know you have one unless the doctor mentions it when you have an internal or you see it yourself during self-examination.

Usually an erosion is best left well alone, since if treatment merely removes the erosion without treating any underlying

hormone imbalance, it will only come back. However if the discharge becomes troublesome or you develop a tendency to vaginal infections you should seek treatment. Conventional treatment consists of burning off the cells or freezing them off. This is not nearly as gruesome as it sounds.

Alternative treatments and self-help

Alternative therapies which treat underlying imbalances are especially useful. Acupuncture, for example, helps 'tune up' the body and removes imbalances. Herbal remedies can be very useful. Golden-seal is according to one medical herbalist 'a marvellous treatment, but it stains everything yellow, and is expensive'. You'd be advised to consult a qualified herbalist rather than trying to treat yourself. Homoeopathic remedies are also useful. Cold hip-baths and practising your pelvic-floor exercises will increase circulation to the area.

Weleda produce a marjoram-balm pessary which is said to be helpful if the erosion becomes infected. It's not available over the counter, so you'd need to consult a herbalist. Any treatment which helps reduce stress, for example meditation, yoga, relaxation techniques and so on is worthwhile, as stress can upset your hormones (see section on periods, page 47).

Infected Bartholin glands

The Bartholin glands are two small rounded glands that lie either side of your vagina and produce mucus when you get sexually aroused. Occasionally one or both of the ducts that normally drain away these secretions becomes blocked or infected, and a small cyst develops. Conventional treatment usually consists of doing nothing, or if the blocked gland becomes troublesome, lancing it to release the fluid

and applying antibiotic cream or ointment.

Alternative treatments

Hot and cold sitz-baths to increase circulation and stimulate glandular activity or hot and cold compresses may be used. A herbalist may recommend a local ointment or lotion, or a solution of goosegrass, or cleavers. Golden-seal again reduces swelling and speeds up healing.

A naturopath may recommend a short fast to rid your body of accumulated poisons, and of course you should get a good wholefood diet.

There are several homoeopathic remedies such as merc sol or belladonna that may be used if the glands are infected and sore. Baryta carb may be recommended if it is merely enlarged but otherwise not causing you any bother. Other remedies include a clay poultice designed to draw out the fluid, and aromatherapy oils such as camomile, thyme, mint and lavender.

AIDS (Acquired Immune Deficiency Syndrome)

Gone is the time when people could believe that AIDS was a disease that only affected homosexual men. The recent campaign has made us all aware that AIDS is now spreading through the heterosexual population too. Some 30,000 people, according to current figures at the time of writing have the AIDS virus — we don't have the exact figures — which means that they are 'antibody positive' to HTLVIII. However, just because you are antibody positive doesn't mean you will necessarily go on to develop the full-blown form of AIDS that you read about in the newspapers. Some 10 per cent *will* develop the most serious form

of the illness, another 10-15 per cent will get minor AIDS-related illness, and the remaining 75 per cent will be unaffected.

AIDS is of course so far incurable by conventional or alternative methods. It is so lethal because it attacks the immune system, paving the way for 'opportunistic' infections, such as a type of meningitis, pneumonia and a type of skin cancer called Kaposi's sarcoma. It can lodge in the brain resulting in nervous system degeneration. If you are pregnant you can pass it on to your unborn baby.

AIDS can lie dormant for a long time after you have first been in contact with it, and it is during this time it may be passed on to others. First symptoms are night sweats, fever, extreme weight loss, lethargy and a general feeling of being unwell, followed by swollen lymph glands and skin blotches.

However with all the panic news articles it is important to put AIDS into perspective. Firstly it's only passed on through the blood or intimate sexual contact. You can't catch it by drinking from the same cup as an AIDS carrier, or by using the same towel as a haemophiliac. Secondly those who do succumb to the illness are often below par physically — that is their immune system is in poor shape to start off with. As we've seen elsewhere in the book, this can have a lot to do with your lifestyle and other factors. The risk is higher if you or your partner sleep around, if your male partner is or has been bi-sexual, or if you or your partner is a drug user or haemophiliac.

Conventional AIDS treatment consists of the use of powerful anti-viral drugs, chemotherapy and Interferon, an anti-cancer drug.

So how can you avoid contracting AIDS, and what does alternative medicine have to offer?

Prevention includes the avoidance of casual sex. Get to know your partner at least a little before leaping into bed with him and don't be afraid to check him out for sexually transmitted diseases — this is where your assertive techniques come in! It's also worth following 'safe sex' guidelines such as using a sheath, and avoiding anal sex. Don't share a razor or hypodermic syringe with anyone else.

Alternative approaches to AIDS focus, as you would expect, on building up the immune system. Previous viruses or bacterial infections, which have involved the use of a lot of antibiotics, may have impaired your immune resistance. Leon Chaitow, in an article in *Here's Health* (March 1986) suggests there is a connection between chronic candida albicans (thrush) and AIDS:

> The frequent use of antibiotics leads to candida proliferation and damage to the normal flora of the bowel (and) also to changes in the control of substances passing from the bowel to the blood-steam. Bowel permeability is altered and this allows undesirable proteins to enter the system, leading to allergies as well as to a drain on immune function.

Diet, as you would expect then, is a mainstay of any alternative approach. A naturopathic regimen of diet and supplements is suggested to rid the body of candida, and boost the body's defences. Professor Jeffrey Bland of the Linus Pauling Institute in the USA recommends large doses of vitamin C and arginine.

Stress reduction techniques, acupuncture to rebalance the body's self-regulating system and herbal medicine are also said to be helpful.

The authors of *AIDS: the deadly epidemic*, describe significant remissions in two sufferers who undertook a holistic pro-gramme of diet, exercise, positive thinking, acupuncture and visualization techniques. Closer to home, AIDS patients at St Mary's Hospital, London are using visualization techniques to try and stimulate healing of their damaged T-cells. In an article in *Homoeopathy Today* (1985/6) a medically qualified homoeopath outlines the possibility of treating AIDS with remedies such as Tuberculin, homoeopathic vaccines such as Carinii for pneumonia and preparations (nosodes) made from the patient's own cancerous tissue or body fluids.

It's only fair to say that neither alternative nor conventional therapies have cracked the AIDS problem, but natural therapies can provide a useful adjunct or even a complete alternative to the more usual treatments. So much research into AIDS is happening at the moment that the information contained in this section may well be outdated by the time you read this. Contact The Terence Higgins Trust or your local health authority for reliable up-to-the-minute facts. The Trust publishes a leaflet, 'Women and AIDS'.

Further information:
AIDS: the deadly epidemic, Graham Hancock and Enver Carim, (Gollancz). The Terence Higgins Trust, BM AIDS, London WC1N 3XX Tel: 01 278 8745.

Pelvic inflammatory disease

Pelvic inflammatory disease (PID) is an umbrella term for a number of pelvic infections. It can be the result of sexually transmitted diseases such as gonorrhoea or chlamydia, or other vaginal infections, birth complications, a septic abortion or be a complication of certain types of IUD. It can cause painful periods. And it's estimated that in 20 per cent of infertile couples the reason for failure to conceive is PID.

Symptoms are low abdominal pain, discharge, a high temperature, pain on intercourse, irregular bleeding and general flu-like symptoms. As the results are potentially so serious you shouldn't try to treat yourself. See a medically qualified homoeopath or herbalist.

Further information:
PID Support Group, c/o Women's Reproductive Rights, 52/54 Featherstone Street, London EC1. Tel: 01-251-6332.

Cystitis

Eight out of ten of us suffer this miserable condition at some time in our lives. Fortunately for most of us it's an isolated event. But for an unlucky few it keeps on coming back and life becomes an endless round of antibiotics, which more often than not result in thrush and the need for further medication.

Symptoms are wanting to empty your bladder frequently, but producing little, burning or stinging when you pass urine, low abdominal pain, or backache, and sometimes bloodstained urine.

In some cases cystitis is caused by straightforward infection. But for about 50 per cent of women, urine analysis shows no signs of bacteria. Triggers are wide-ranging — they can include sex, alcohol, tea and coffee, too much sugar in the diet, heat and cold, wearing tight clothing, prolapse, chemicals in soap, bubble baths, the swimming-pool or spermicides — and that's just a few. Some of us experience minor cystitis just before a period.

Orthodox treatment

This consists of antibiotics, and sometimes a preparation to rebalance the pH level of the urine called Potassium Citrate (Pot. Cit.), plus advice to drink plenty of fluids and to rest. Very occasionally women may be given a 'urethral stretch' which seems to alleviate symptoms for some.

But about one in ten women who experience repeated attacks resist antibiotic treatment, and for them the medics have coined the term 'urethral syndrome.' So what has alternative medicine to offer? And is there anything you can do to help yourself?

Self-help and alternative treatment

As you will realize by now, stress is one of the foundations of many illnesses from an alternative viewpoint, and sure enough, stress seems to make cystitis worse. There are a number of things you can do to help prevent full-blown cystitis coming on, and alternative therapies are also very successful in treating it.

Both herbalism and homoeopathy are helpful in cystitis. Apis is a remedy which is often especially useful. Naturopathic treatment concentrates on diet. You may be given dolomite which helps some women.

Clinical ecology is coming up with some interesting methods, based on the idea that cystitis is caused by food allergy. They consist of giving injections or drops of small quantities of the offending foods well diluted.

Aromatherapy, consisting of compresses and massage as well as warm baths can be helpful: cedarwood and pine may be useful.

Osteopathy or chiropractic may be able to iron out any anatomical problems that may predispose you to cystitis. For instance, a retroverted uterus may press on your bladder causing urine retention.

Acupuncture also works very well in cases of cystitis. While biochemic tissue salts can be a first line in an emergency: Ferr Phos, Kali Mur, Kali Phos and Mag Phos are the suggested remedies, depending on your symptoms.

To prevent an attack

● Eat a good wholefood diet.

● Drink three to four pints of liquid a day, but lay off too much tea and coffee. Herb teas and mineral waters are better.

● Don't hang on if you want to empty your bladder, go to the toilet regularly.

● Don't use vaginal deodorants, bubble baths, talc and perfumed soap.

● Pay attention to hygiene. Wash after opening your bowels using plain cool water.

● Wipe your bottom from front to back to prevent germs from the anus entering your urinary tract.

● You and your partner should wash before sex.

● Empty your bladder before and as soon after sex as you can. Wash your genital area too by pouring cool water over it so as to flush out any germs that may have entered while you were making love.

● Avoid love-making positions that put pressure on the bladder. Positions where you are on top, or your partner enters from behind may be better than the good old missionary.

• Don't make love until you are well-aroused, so as to avoid vaginal dryness. If for any reasons your natural secretions are scanty (for example after the menopause) use aloe vera gel for lubrication.

• Practise pelvic-floor exercises to generally strengthen the area.

• Avoid tight jeans and knickers and go for cotton underwear. Watch what you wash your underwear in — no biological washing powders.

If you develop an attack

• At the very first twinge increase your fluid intake. Drink half a pint of water every 20 minutes for three hours.

• Take a teaspoon of bicarbonate of soda in water every other hour on the first day, less often after that, and don't continue for more than three days. This tastes quite foul and may be more acceptable if you mix in a little fruit juice which makes it fizz, or runny honey. Bicarbonate of soda shouldn't be taken if you suffer from high blood pressure. If this applies to you, or you simply find it too nasty to drink, try vitamin C tablets instead — 3g a day over the course of four days.

• A herbalist recommends a tea made of equal quantities of meadowsweet and buchu leaf to be drunk as often as you like.

• Stay warm. Place a hot water bottle wrapped in a towel against your back or pelvic area.

• Steer clear of coffee, tea, alcohol and anything spicy.

• Avoid meat, shellfish, anchovies, sardines, sugar, prunes, lettuce, carrots, green beans and spinach. All these can make your urine acid and increase stinging.

• Drink barley water to soothe inflammation.

• Eat leeks! They are alkaline and act both as an antiseptic and diuretic.

• If you do have to have antibiotics make sure you get plenty of vitamin C, since they rob your body of this vitamin. Eat plenty of yogurt to rebalance your system, or take acidophilus tablets.

Benign breast disease

Cancer has such a high profile that it's hardly surprising that many of us panic at the slightest thing going wrong with our breasts. Do bear in mind that 75 per cent of breast lumps are absolutely harmless. Especially if you are under 40 most breast problems are due to what doctors call benign breast disease.

Lumps and bumps

Many of us experience tender, lumpy breasts just before a period, especially during our teens and in the years preceding the menopause. The lumpiness, which seems to be a result of the way the body reacts to its own hormones, passes off once your period is over, and is nothing to worry about.

As you get older, more definite lumps or cysts may appear. Fibrocystic disease is the rather vague umbrella term sometimes used to describe these. Occasionally the doctor will drain the cyst to make sure it isn't malignant — more often than not it's safe to leave it alone. A lump that is hard to pin down is a fibroadenoma, sometimes called a 'breast mouse' because it is so mobile. Simple reassurance that it isn't cancer is all that's usually necessary, or the lump may be removed.

Other less common signs of benign breast disease are nipple discharge, nipple retraction and skin problems like eczema. Nipple discharge though alarming is not always serious. It may be white, creamy, green, yellow, clear or even bloodstained. It's usually the result of a non-cancerous lump in the ducts (ductal papilloma). Surgery will usually be advised to rule out the possibility that the lump is cancerous.

The usual orthodox approach to benign breast disease is hormones, analgesics, and as already described in some cases, surgery.

What has alternative medicine got to offer?
A broad based dietary approach can help enormously. There's quite a lot of evidence accruing that benign breast disease may be a result of allergy. Excess caffeine seems to play a part, so cut coffee, tea and cola-type drinks if you are prone.

Evening primrose oil, already described under PMS, will reduce swelling and pain for many women. Homoeopathy and herbalism can help correct hormonal imbalances.

On a practical level, wear a good supporting bra, and get plenty of exercise to stimulate circulation to the breasts. Yoga may be especially helpful — try the bow and cobra postures (page 50). For others consult your yoga teacher.

Perhaps the most exciting new approach comes from the USA. It's thought that in benign breast disease the body is sensitized in some way to it's own hormones. Homoeopathic dosages of oestrogen and progesterone have been given to some women with what one practitioner describes as 'a number of useful outcomes.' The treatment isn't widely available as yet, but if you are interested consult a clinical ecologist.

The symptoms of benign breast disease and cancer can be the same, so if you do develop a breast problem, don't delay seeing your doctor or a medically qualified alternative practitioner. But, as I said at the outset, the vast majority of these problems aren't usually serious. Don't be afraid to ask your therapist exactly what is wrong — for your own peace of mind.

Cancer

In this section I want to look at the main cancers that affect women, what you can expect in the way of orthodox treatment, and how you can help yourself. Finally I'll be looking at the role alternative medicine has to play.

Can you prevent cancer?

Cancer prevention involves following three simple rules:

● As far as possible avoid exposure to cancer causing-substances such as tobacco, chemicals at work, additives and so on.

● Adopt a healthy lifestyle — the tips for staying healthy (Part One, page 13) are useful here. A diet rich in vitamin A is said to be especially useful.

● See your doctor if you develop any of the following:

☐ a sore that doesn't heal

☐ an unusual lump or thickening

☐ unusual bleeding or discharge

☐ a change in a wart or mole, for example itchiness, bleeding

☐ difficulty in swallowing or persistent indigestion

☐ persistent hoarseness or a cough

☐ a change in your usual bowel habits

Breast cancer

Breast cancer. The very words make many of us quail. It's hardly surprising. One in twelve women develop breast cancer. And the disease is still the number one killer of women aged between 35 and 54. Despite new forms of treatment, the five year survival rate for breast cancer remains pegged at around 50 per cent, regardless of how many check-ups you have had, and regardless of treatment. What's more, this figure has barely shifted in the last 50 years. And when it comes to treatment, there is an amazing amount of disagreement among doctors, so that the treatment you receive is as likely to do with where you live and the views of your doctor, as to do with the type of cancer you have.

But all is not complete doom and gloom. A recent conference at the King's Fund centre, held in October 1986, has come up with a consensus statement designed to iron out variations in orthodox treatment. While on the alternative front there are a number of promising developments. Finally, new research into the role of the immune system in disease looks set to build a bridge between orthodox and alternative approaches to treatment.

Because breast cancer is so common it's

well worth thinking about it *now*, then if you should ever need to, you will be in a better position to make the choices that are right for you.

So who gets breast cancer? Is there anything you can do to reduce your chances of developing it? And if you are diagnosed as having breast cancer what sort of help is available?

Risk factors for breast cancer
You stand a higher chance of getting breast cancer if you fall into one or more of the following groups

☐ You have no children

☐ You have your first child over the age of 25 (some experts say 30)

☐ You began your periods early

☐ You have a late menopause

☐ Your mother, grandmother, sister or other close female relative has had breast cancer

☐ You are overweight

☐ You have a history of cancer in the other breast or elsewhere in the body.

You'll see the factors that put you at an increased risk of developing breast cancer in the box above. That's not to say that if you have any of these risk factors you are bound to get the disease. But if you do come into any of these categories, it will certainly pay you to be extra careful and well informed, in order to avoid unnecessary

additional risks, and so that you can seek early treatment if you do get it.

How can I tell?
The incidence of breast cancer increases with age. The commonest symptom is a lump or deformity in the breast. Look out for any dimpling or a retracted nipple that isn't normal for you — especially if the nipple is pulled in all round, rather than just in a strip across the nipple. Contrary to conventional wisdom, pain *can* be a symptom of breast cancer, especially if you are past the menopause. Nipple discharge is also a sign, and very occasionally there are no symptoms at all. That's not to say that any of these symptoms *is* breast cancer. As the section on benign breast disease showed, all these symptoms can also indicate far less serious problems. Even so, you'd be wise to consult your doctor or a medically qualified alternative practitioner if you do experience any of them.

The commonest place to find a lump is the upper, outer quarter of your breast, followed by the upper, inner quarter, or the underside of the breast.

See your doctor if you develop any of the following:

☐ Change in the shape or size of one of your breasts

☐ Puckering or dimpling of the skin

☐ Enlarged veins

☐ Lump or thickening of breast tissue

☐ Nipple discharge

☐ Retracted nipple

☐ Change in skin texture or rash on the nipple

☐ Swelling of the upper arm, armpit or above your breast

☐ Non-cyclical breast pain

Diagnosis

The doctor will examine your breasts and in six cases out of ten will be able to hazard a fair guess if the cause of the problem is breast cancer. You may then be sent for mammography (a special breast X-ray). If cancer is suspected, a biopsy, which involves taking a sample of the diseased tissue, will confirm diagnosis. This may be done by aspiration (when a small sample is sucked out through a fine needle), or by removing a cone of tissue or a small part of the lump. Further investigtions to ascertain the type of cancer and how far it may have spread can include blood tests, X-rays and sometimes an estimation of liver function.

It can be frightening to be told you have breast cancer. Do bear in mind that breast cancer is not just a disease that woman die from. Many live with it for many years. And though neither alternative nor orthodox therapies can claim to have cracked breast cancer, it is something that can often be controlled. A pamphlet produced by the Manchester Well Woman Group, *Thinking about breast cancer,* makes the following point: 'The most important thing is that women who want to do so can keep some control over what is happening to them.' The more you know about treatment options, the more you can co-operate and decide on

the sort of treatment that will suit you best.

Orthodox treatment

At one time anyone diagnosed as having breast cancer would automatically expect to have her breast removed. However studies have shown that mastectomy or more extensive breast surgery, as opposed to just removing the lump, do *not* lead to longer survival. (Though the risk of the cancer recurring in the affected breast is higher if the lump alone is removed.) This risk can be reduced by follow-up treatment with radiotherapy.

Your options will depend on the type of cancer and whether there is any evidence that it has spread elsewhere in your body.

In early breast cancer, that is where the lump is less than 5cm in diameter and there is no evidence that it has spread (metastasised), surgery is the first line of treatment. This can take several forms:

● Lumpectomy — the lump and a small area of surrounding tissue are removed.

● Partial mastectomy — a larger part of the breast is removed.

● Total mastectomy — the whole of your breast and the lymph glands are removed but the underlying muscles are left.

● Radical mastectomy — where the whole of the breast, the lymph glands under the arm and the underlying muscles are removed. This is much less often performed today than in the past.

Where there are several lumps or a large part of the breast is affected, mastectomy may be the best surgical treatment, or you may prefer it to prevent the chance of cancer occurring again in the same breast, or if you want to avoid radiotherapy.

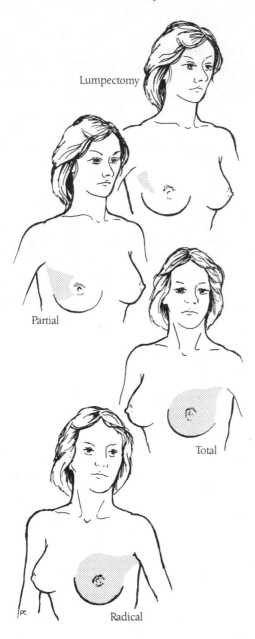

Lumpectomy

Partial

Total

Radical

Figure 10: Types of mastectomy.

Back-up treatment (adjuvant therapy)
This is aimed at wiping out any remaining cancer cells.

Radiotherapy — a carefully controlled dose of radiation is aimed at the cancer site. The snag is the X-rays can't discriminate between cancer cells and non-cancer cells, and the treatment has several unpleasant side-effects such as exhaustion, nausea, skin soreness, that usually come on after two to three weeks. What's more, the body can only take so much radiation, which has the effect of lowering the body's immune defences. Sometimes radioactive metal wire implants are used to provide booster doses of radiation to the bed of the lump.

Chemotherapy (drug treatment) — Drugs that kill off the cells as they divide (cytotoxic) are given, the idea being that as cancer cells divide very rapidly they can be killed off without destroying the healthy cells. The biggest drawback is the side-effects, which include nausea, hair loss, loss of appetite and taste, weakness, numbness of the fingers and toes and anxiety. Combinations of cytotoxic drugs reduce the risk of death over a five year period by about 9 per cent, for certain groups of women. However, the treatment is less useful for women over 50, and the costs and benefits need to be carefully weighed up in each particular case. New 'targeted' cytotoxic drugs designed to bind only on to cancer cells themselves offer the promise of a way around some of the problems of side-effects. But these are not yet available.

Hormone treatment
Tumours of the sort that depend on oestrogen to grow can be treated with an

anti-oestrogen drug called Tamoxifen. This is usually the first line of treatment if you are over 70 or have problems such as heart disease which might make an operation risky. Alternatively, Tamoxifen may be given for a couple of years as a back-up to surgery or other treatment. The reduced rates of relapse in women over fifty seem to make this a worthwhile treatment for those of us in this age group. Side effects seem to be relatively few, they include hot flushes, nausea and headache. However, it's only fair to say that no one yet knows what the long term effects of such treatment may be.

Treating the ovaries

As I've already said, many breast cancers are oestrogen dependent. It would seem to follow that preventing the ovaries, which produce most of the body's oestrogen, from working, might have an effect of reducing the tumour. This is occasionally done either by removing the ovaries (oophorectomy), or by destroying their action by radiation. This seems to help in women past the menopause. If you are younger than this such a procedure will cause early menopause, and an increased likelihood of heart disease, since the female hormones protect women against heart problems.

Decision time

You may be the sort of person who is happy to hand over to your doctor and let him decide on treatment, in which case fair enough. On the other hand, several studies suggest that counselling and understanding can do much to reduce anxiety and distress. Try to find out as much you can about your cancer, what stage it is at, and how far it may have spread, as well as your specialist's favoured treatment methods. Discuss possible side effects. It can be hard to think straight, and remember what questions you want to ask when you are feeling worried, so take along a friend or partner and make a list of questions.

Remember, many lumps have been there for several years before discovery. A couple of weeks' delay while you explore the pros and cons of different forms of treatment isn't going to make any difference to the success of your treatment.

Where cancer has spread

If your cancer has spread, treatment will be aimed at controlling symptoms, preventing it recurring elsewhere and keeping you in as good health as possible. Treatment again will depend on your age, where the cancer is, the length of time between initial treatment and spread. Hormone treatments alone may be offered, chemotherapy, hormone injections and radiotherapy can all be part of the treatment.

Life after mastectomy

For most of us our breasts are very important. In a world where our mammaries are used to sell everything from newspapers to cars, it's hardly surprising that we should see them as symbols of our sexuality. We feed our babies with them and we get sexual pleasure from them, so the loss or disfigurement of a breast may lead to deep feelings of loss. Complete removal of the breast, as I said earlier, is much less common today. If you do have this done it's important not to bottle up your feelings. Talk them over with a nurse, doctor, skilled counsellor or friend. Give yourself time to grieve and expect to feel angry, depressed and confused. It's all part of the mourning process.

Breast reconstruction

The words breast reconstruction can make your body sound a bit like a building site.

An implant can be put in at the time of the original operation or later, or you may be offered a prosthesis. Where the cancer is small and doesn't appear to have spread, this can be very successful, and may help you regain a sense of identity. However, some women feel that the rush to recreate what was there is a way of avoiding coming to terms with the illness, and seeing its meaning. They argue that in a world where women are often judged purely on appearance and sexual attractiveness, treating breast cancer as merely a cosmetic problem that can be put right as simply as a facelift, is a way of denying the importance of the experience. That's not to say that it might not be right for some of us, but do give the matter some careful thought before leaping at the chance of prosthesis.

Future check-ups
You'll be given regular check-ups to make sure all is still well after initial treatment. It's natural to feel worried, and to find all sorts of lumps and bumps before going for a check-up. Taking along a friend, and being open about your feelings will help.

Genital cancers

Cancer can occur in the vulva and vagina, cervix (neck of the womb), the body of the uterus, ovaries and Fallopian tubes. Of these, cervical cancer is by far the most common, and cancer of the Fallopian tube the least. Cancer of the uterus usually occurs between the ages of 50 and 60, and you are at greater risk of developing it if you have diabetes or are overweight. Cancer of the ovaries also occurs mainly in older women. Cancer of the vulva and vagina are relatively rare.

Cervical cancer
Cancer of the cervix is commonest between

the ages of 45 and 50, but recently the age at which it strikes has been creeping down. Normal cervical cells undergo certain pre-cancerous changes, and if the condition can be nipped in the bud, treatment is virtually one hundred per cent successful. If it progresses, treatment is much more difficult. Because of this, the traditional focus has been on detecting these changes early on by means of a Pap test, otherwise known as a cervical smear.

Smear-test
A smear is a simple painless test, in which a few cells are taken from the neck of your womb and analysed for pre-cancerous changes.

In Scandinavia the incidence of cervical cancer has been cut by half following the introduction of regular smear-testing. In Canada the death rate has dropped by a staggering 90 per cent. In the UK however, though deaths from cervical cancer have dropped overall, its incidence in younger age groups is increasing. What's more, this type of cancer seems to progress faster than the type found in older age groups.

One reason is that our present smear programme is patchy and inadequate. Many women who are most at risk are falling through the screening net. Not all G.P.s carry out smear-tests. There is no central recall system to tell you when a smear is due, and women are rarely notified of results. If you don't have regular contact with the health services, for instance if your children are older, or you don't attend a family planning clinic, you may well miss out. This could be the very time you are most at risk. At the time of writing the BMA have just issued a plan of action that they recommend the government should take up, including 3-yearly smear-tests for women aged twenty and over, (or younger if their sex life began earlier), proper recall facilities, and better local organization of the system. They also advise a massive health education programme to help ensure that those who are at high risk get tested. It's to be hoped that by the time you read this the government will have taken some sort of action.

How often should I have a smear?
Expert opinion is divided. It used to be thought that every five years should be the recommended time between tests. Today experts are more likely to suggest that women over 35 attend every two years, while those in a high risk group should have a smear every year.

What if I have a positive smear?
It can be frightening to be told your smear is positive. Remember — it doesn't always mean you have cancer. It usually means that some of the cells have changed in such a way that could lead to cancer if they continued to undergo such changes. We don't know how often cells do change and return to normal. But it's a fact that often the cells will revert to their usual state. Regular smear-testing may be all that is required.

More severe changes in the cells will be treated. You'll be given a coposcopy (examination of the cervix with a microscope) to see the extent of changes. The cells will then be destroyed using laser, freezing them off, or carrying out a cone biopsy, in which a small part of the cervix is removed under anaesthetic. After a cone biopsy you'll experience some bleeding. Your cervix may be weaker after the operation, and if you go on to become

pregnant you may need a special stitch to avoid miscarriage.

Incidentally if you have an abnormal smear you don't have to give up sex. It can't make the condition worse, and you can't pass it on to your partner. Making love can be a valuable source of comfort when you are feeling worried.

Abnormal smears are graded from one to three. CIN (cervical intra-epithelial neoplasis) 1 smears will be repeated after three months to see if the condition has progressed — in many cases the smear will have returned to normal and you are in the clear. CIN 2 and 3 smears will be referred to a gynaecologist for treatment.

Am I at risk?
Women who are at greatest risk of developing cervical cancer are:

☐ Those who have had several sex partners, or whose partner has had several sex partners.

☐ Those who smoke or, occasionally, whose partners smoke.

☐ Those who have genital warts (HMPV) or whose partner has genital warts.

☐ Those with a large family, especially if you started your family early.

☐ Those with husbands who work in 'dirty' or dusty jobs such as miners, metal workers, leather workers, or those who work on machines or with certain chemicals, or textiles.

In the rare event that cancer has progressed further than this, treatment is by surgery, radiotherapy, and in more advanced cases chemotherapy.

Orthodox treatment for genital cancers consists of surgery, plus chemotherapy and/or radiotherapy as a back up.

The alternative approach to cancer

It's clear that orthodox medicine doesn't have all the answers where cancer is concerned. And while conventional treatment is undoubtedly effective in treating some forms of cancer such as blood, skin, lymph gland, testes and cervix, if carried out early enough — in other cases treatment is distinctly hit and miss. Breast cancer is an obvious example, where as already observed, survival rates have remained virtually the same for years despite advances in treatment and detection. Surgery and radiotherapy may kill cancer cells, but they allow little scope for the body to heal itself, and as we've seen may have unpleasant side-effects.

An increasing body of evidence suggests that all of us have cancer cells in our bodies at times during our lives. In most cases our immune systems swing into action to fight off the disease before it has a chance to take hold. For some reason in people who develop the full-blown illness this fails to happen. The observation that those who have undergone severely stressful experiences such as bereavement or divorce have lowered immune resistance, and are more likely to fall prey to cancer offers some valuable clues as to why some people should be at risk. Resistance may also be lowered by diet, genetics, hormonal or environmental factors.

Preventive tips

● Barrier methods of contraception such as the sheath or the cap are thought to offer greater protection against abnormal cervical changes. (One study showed that in women with positive smears whose partners started using a sheath the cells went back to normal).

● Immunity can be lower as a result of stress or lack of vitamins. Concentrate on stress reduction techniques, yoga, meditation, relaxation and exercise. And make sure you get a good diet.

● You and your partner should keep your sexual organs clean. It's a good idea for the man to wash before sex.

● If you or your partner develop genital warts, herpes or chlamydia, make sure you get treatment, and make a point of having regular smear-tests.

See your doctor if

☐ You develop any abnormal bleeding from the vagina.

☐ You experience an unusual or offensive vaginal discharge.

☐ You suffer unexplained weight-loss or a swollen abdomen.

☐ You develop an ulcer on your genitals that fails to heal, or any unusual lump or bump.

Most alternative practitioners take the view that cancer is not merely a disease of the cells, but a disease of the whole person. This approach is summed up by the director of the charity New Approaches to Cancer who told me 'Our approach to cancer is that cancer is a deeper problem within a person and unless the deeper problem is resolved then the cancer will more than likely appear in another area if only treated by conventional methods.' The alternative approach, as you'd expect is geared to the whole person, rather than to treatment of any particular form of cancer. What's more, it doesn't distinguish between male and female cancers, though as the director of New Approaches to Cancer says again: One aspect of our approach that we would see very applicable, particularly to breast cancer, would be that of emotional trauma, either acute through loss or separation, or chronic through non-existent or disturbed relationships.

Because alternative approaches to cancer set out from a different starting point to conventional medicine, it's very difficult to compare one treatment against the other. Holistic G.P. Dr Patrick Pietroni writes in an article in the medical journal, *Cancer Topics* (Sept/Oct 1986): 'It would be fair to say that there is no objective evidence as yet that any of these techniques add to longevity for any one group of patients. However, *nearly all studies remark on the improvement in quality-of-life and the relationships surrounding the patient, his (sic) family and advisors.*'

So, if you want to undertake alternative treatment for cancer, it would be wise not to undergo it with the view that it will *cure* you. What it can do is to help you to sort out the meaning of your cancer for you personally, and perhaps alleviate symptoms.

Incidentally, a trial is now taking place at the Bristol Cancer Help Centre to compare 5 year survival rates of women with breast cancer from orthodox and alternative treatment, so we may soon have some more definite answers to the question: 'Does alternative medicine work for cancer?'

The immune system link

Once again the immune system and its relation to other parts of us is the lynchpin of the alternative approach. An increasing body of clinical evidence lends weight to the suggestion that stress lowers the body's immune resistance and so encourages cancer growth.

The main aim of all alternative treatments is to boost your body's defences by various methods. Cancer being the end result of a long degenerative process you shouldn't try to go it completely alone. Find a sympathetic practitioner and let your doctor know.

What can I expect?

The main lines of attack from an alternative position are to look at diet, and the influence of mind and spirit on the body. Homoeopathy, herbal medicine and acupuncture also all have something to offer.

Is there a cancer personality?

Several studies now show a possible connection between cancer and personality. Holistic practitioner Laurence LeShan lists the following characteristics that he has found to be common to cancer patients:

● Unsettled childhood.

● Low opinion of yourself.

● Unsatisfactory relationship with your parents.

- No creative outlets.

- Keeping a tight lid on your emotions.

- A defeatist attitude.

- Loss of an important relationship.

It could be said that, in our society, almost anyone will have experienced one or more of these. And many people would argue that such a classification leads to victim-blaming and guilt. Nevertheless, loss does have a crucial part to play in depression as you'll see in the mind-body section. Women in particular experience loss in a particular way, because so often they see themselves in relation to others around them, rather than as autonomous beings.

According to the studies just mentioned cancer patients are of a particular personality type. Basically they are 'nice' people. The argument goes that when such a person experiences a major loss, the body's immune system becomes depressed and fails to cope with cancer cells. A study at King's College Hospital, London showed that the 5-year survival rate amongst women with breast cancer depended critically upon attitude. Patients with a fighting spirit, or those who denied that they had cancer and just got on with life, survived more than twice as long as those who simply gave in. A large dose of optimism, or refusal to give in, apparently stimulates the body's antibody system.

It's only fair to say that such research is still in its infancy, and not surprisingly many orthodox oncologists (cancer specialists) dismiss it completely. One leading cancer specialist writing in the doctor's magazine *Pulse* writes: 'Cancer of the breast has an unpredictable course; at one extreme patients may die within a month of diagnosis and at the other, patients with advanced disease may live for many years. By carefully selecting the type of case, evidence can be accumulated that any treatment can prolong life.' However, the same specialist is forced to concede that much orthodox medicine retains practices that are completely unscientific as well as being potentially dangerous and invasive.

Studies are currently being carried out in Manchester and London to examine these ideas further, so we may soon have a more definite answer to the question: 'Is there a cancer personality?'

Visualization
This is a technique pioneered in the USA by Carl and Stephanie Simonton which uses a mixture of breathing, relaxation, meditation, hypnosis and positive thinking. The idea is that you are encouraged to think of the cancer cells as 'weak and confused' and to focus on the stronger healthy cells in your body fighting them off. To give you a flavour of what this involves I quote a passage from the book *Love, Medicine and Miracles* (Rider) by U.S. doctor Bernie S. Siegel: 'I told my body to be well. I told my immunological system to protect me. I looked at my brain, my bones, my liver and my lungs every night. I felt them and told them to be free of cancer. I watched my blood flowing strongly. I told the wound to heal quickly and the area around it to be clean. I told my other breast to behave, because it's the only one my husband and I have left. I still tell my body and mind every night, "I reject cancer. I reject cancer." '

Such visualization techniques are enormously flexible. You can use any images that suit you. You don't have to use the language of attack. In fact, as Bernie S. Siegel points out, the 'war model' of cancer may in fact be inappropriate since the cancer cells are your own cells gone astray. Imagining your white cells engulfing the cancer cells, or eating them may well be more appealing images, especially for women.

The meaning of cancer

An important part of the alternative approach to cancer is to help people to discover the meaning that cancer has for them. Illness, and cancer is no exception, can make it easier to say no to things we don't want to do, or to escape from the demands placed on us by others. This may be especially significant for women who both have to conform to the often contradictory and unrealistic expectations placed on them by others, as well as finding it difficult to say no. Illness can be a way of getting the love of nurturance that we may feel unable to ask for in any other way. It's reasoned that once you know what psychological needs the illness is serving you can begin to satisfy them in different ways. Ann Oakley, whom I quoted earlier, vividly recreates the meaning that cancer of the mouth had for her in her book, *Taking it like a Woman* (Flamingo): 'To have a cancer in my mouth was a direct attack on my identity. Given the importance of words in my work I needed my mouth, not primarily to speak but to think in words, to write. It was where I lived. It was the source of my vitality, my creativity . . . and also a site of my sexuality. Because of this, one of the first things Robin did when the diagnosis of cancer was made was to kiss me.'

At the Bristol Cancer Help Centre, and other places using alternative approaches to cancer, a lot of emphasis is laid on cancer as a 'transformational experience' that can change your whole way of experiencing life.

Ann Oakley again: 'It became clear to me that living in the present does have to do with knowing who one is, but that it also has to do with appreciating that timelessness denied by the modern world in its preoccupation with superficial change and senescence, with making a friend of eternity.'

Finally, although reports of 'cures' are purely anecdotal, as Patrick Pietroni points out in the article mentioned earlier: 'Those few anecdotal reports on spontaneous regression in cancer all describe what has been termed "a dramatic existential shift" . . . involving a resurgence of hope, together with an alternation in belief system and acceptance of responsibility for the process of healing and recovery.'

The diet connection

If you've read this far you won't be surprised to discover that the other mainstay of the alternative approach to cancer is diet. A report by two orthodox oncologists in 1981 laid a third of all cancers at the door of diet. Many alternative practitioners would put the figure much higher.

The key, certainly where women's cancers are concerned, may lie in some connection between hormones and diet. Breast cancer is far more common in countries where fat plays a large part in diet, for example. Oestrogen has an important role in female cancers of all kinds. Breast cancer rates are higher in women who began their periods early and who had a late menopause, and who therefore have high levels of circulating oestrogen for longer. It's known too that oestrogen is produced by body fat. A recent study published in the journal *Cancer* reports that women with breast cancer have higher levels of oestradiol (a form of oestrogen) in their bloodstreams compared with a control group. What's more, a report which appeared in the *American Journal of Clinical Nutrition* in 1984 points to the significance of diet in length of menstrual cycle. White women fed on a meatless diet had fewer periods. The report suggests we should look at the possibilities of using vegetarian diets in post-menopausal cancer patients.

Women with positive smears have been discovered to have diets containing less than 30mg of vitamin C a day. This could help explain why women who smoke seem to be at a higher risk of developing cervical cancer, as smoking robs the body of vitamin C (as does the Pill). Low levels of vitamin C have also been associated with breast cancer.

Other studies have linked low levels of vitamin A and beta-carotene, a type of vitamin A, to the development of cancer. The Hunza tribe of northern Pakistan who eat a diet high in B_{17} found in dried apricots, the kernels of cherries, apricots, apple pips and so on are remarkably free of cancer. Though, so far as I know, no one has studied the social factors in this community, which may go some way to explaining their apparent resistance to the disease. A study in the *British Journal of Cancer* has shown that women with early cancer of the cervix had less beta-carotene in their bloodstream than a control group. Vitamin E and the mineral selenium have also been implicated in the prevention of cancer.

As always, the story is far from clear-cut, and we don't yet know how these nutrients may serve to protect against cancer, nor how useful they are in treating it. Vitamin A, for example, may block the effect of carcinogens in the breast and reproductive system, and may also prevent the body from converting cancer-causing chemicals into toxins.

As you would expect fibre too seems to play a large part in preventing cancer. A study carried out in the Bristol area looking at the incidence of bowel cancer and the intake of fibre and fat found that those with cancer consumed less fibre and more sugar than a healthy control group. This can perhaps be explained by the fact that fibre binds cancer-causing substances in the body and speeds their progress through the gut.

One other point that is perhaps less often mentioned in dietary studies is the effect how we eat our food has on us. Patrick Pietroni in the article quoted earlier describes a study carried out in Ohio on rabbits which found a 60 per cent reduction in the incidence of arterial problems in a group of rabbits fed a high fat diet: 'This group of rabbits were being fed by a different laboratory technician who insisted on taking each rabbit out of its cage, calming and stroking it before it was fed its high fat diet.'

Is it too fantastic to reason that humans too might benefit from a calmer state of mind at mealtimes? Might this explain why some people, in spite of an apparently poor diet don't go on to develop cancer or heart disease?

Diets for the treatment of cancer
Dietary treatments for cancer include a whole range of approaches which include fasting, detoxification, the use of supplements, injections of laetrile (an enzyme found in apricot kernels which is thought to explain why the Hunzas are resistant to cancer) and coffee enemas.

Two of the most famous dietary regimes are the Gerson diet and Bristol Diet, developed at the Bristol Cancer Help Centre. Briefly, the Gerson diet works on the principle that cancer patients have low immune response and generalized tissue damage, especially of the liver. When cancer is eliminated by whatever method of treatment, poisonous wastes appear in the bloodstream that eventually destroy the body, unless they are disposed of. The diet aims to regenerate the body and to stimulate its self-healing mechanisms. It's an extremely rigorous regime which includes no tap water, smoking or alcohol, and women aren't allowed to use make up. However, a five-year trial carried out in Australia of patients where cancer had spread to the liver shows several unexpected partial remissions.

The Bristol Cancer Help Centre Diet adheres to the following principles:

● No animal products.

● Mainly raw food.

● No junk food.

● No coffee or tea. One glass of wine or a measure of spirits are allowed each day, as they are thought to stimulate the production of prostaglandin B_{17}.

● No salt.

● The inclusion of sprouted seeds which are rich in B_{17}. (There's been some recent controversy about this since sprouted alfalfa has been found to contain substances that supress the immune system. Adherents of the Gerson regime have now abandoned sprouted seeds altogether, but the Bristol Centre still uses them.

● Vitamin supplements of A, B, C, and E. (But not vitamin E for hormone-dependent breast cancers.)

● Mineral supplements of magnesium, potassium, calcium, zinc, selenium.

As always then, the message seems to be to cut down on fat, sugar, processed foods and step up your intake of fresh foods, fibre, vitamins and minerals.

Further information:
Of course it's impossible in a book this size to do full justice to the complexities of the various dietary methods. If you are interested in finding out more I suggest you read, *The Bristol Programme*, by Penny Brown, (Century), and *The Bristol Recipe Book*, (Century).
Alternatively, contact New Approaches to Cancer, c/o Seekers Trust, Addington Park, Maidstone, Kent, ME19 5BL, who will be able to put you in touch with a medically qualified practitioner interested in dietary methods.

Alternative cancer treatment

● Diet.

● Relaxation.

● Yoga, T'ai chi.

● Megavitamin therapy.

● Counselling and/or psycho-therapy.

● Exercise.

● Avoidance of chemicals in the environment e.g. aerosol sprays.

● Creative expression e.g. art therapy, dance therapy.

● Acupuncture or TENS.

● Spiritual healing.

● Meditation/Visualization techniques.

Other alternative cancer treatments
These include the use of iscador (mistletoe) in homoeopathic doses or herbal preparations. Other herbal treatments for cancer include those that work on the liver such as burdock, blue flag, yellow dock, on the lymphatic system, such as cleavers, echinacea and poke root, and other herbs such as sweet violet.

TENS and acupuncture can play a part in pain relief, and spiritual healing is an important part of treatment in alternative cancer centres.

You may want to undertake alternative treatment in conjunction with orthodox medicine, either as a preliminary to surgery and the rest, or as a back-up. Only orthodox practitioners can prescribe specific cancer treatments, of course, and it's here that we come up against the difference of approach between orthodox and alternative therapists again. Most alternative practitioners would claim not to be treating the cancer, but the whole person.

Before I end this chapter — a word of warning. Do remember that if you have cancer your body has broken down in a big

way and has more than likely been weakened further by aggressive surgery or drugs. Any alternative treatment you undergo is going to take time — and no one can expect miracles. Inevitably many people with cancer aren't cured, any more than they would be by orthodox methods. However, a large number who have undergone alternative therapy testify to the improved 'quality' of their lives. Perhaps I should end this chapter with two quotations that I hope sum up the spirit of what I have written. The first comes from a cancer patient writing in the British magazine *Spare Rib*, the second are the words of American feminist Audre Lorde whose *The Cancer Journals*, (Sheba) well repays a read: 'If we keep fit and survive long after the medicos think we can — what does it matter which treatment worked?' 'I would never have chosen this path, but I am very glad to be who I am, here.'

Further information:
Women's National Cancer Control Campaign, 1 South Audley Street, London W1Y 5DQ.

Women's Health Information Centre, 52/54 Featherstone Street, London EC1.

Mental health

The size of the problem
Doctors' surgeries are crammed with people who are visiting not because of any physical condition, but because of emotional disturbance. Of course, such disturbances can affect people physically, as the section on stress showed. In the course of 20 years, three-quarters of women and half of men in this country will find themselves seeing the doctor with a mental health problem.

Of these women are twice as likely to complain of depression. If you are a married woman you are more likely to suffer from anxiety than a married man. And two-thirds of agoraphobics are women. Why?

Anxiety and depression are often the end products of stress overload, and as we saw in section one, there are many aspects of women's lives that lay them open to stress. Women are encouraged to express their feelings more openly than men. Whereas a man who is feeling depressed or anxious may be inclined to take refuge in excessive drinking or sex, or keep a stiff upper lip, women are more likely to make their way to the doctor's surgery. What's more, in our jobs as mothers and wives, we are more likely to have direct contact with the medical services, so this may seem the obvious place to seek help for emotional problems.

Depression is often sparked off by a loss of some kind — perhaps the loss of a job, a partner or even a cherished belief. That's not to say that everyone who experiences any sort of loss automatically becomes depressed. And of course a period of depression and mourning can be a perfectly natural and appropriate response to certain aspects of life, for instance following a marriage break up. But there are some factors that make women more vulnerable. Joanna Ryan points out in a pamphlet on *Feminism and Therapy*, written for the Women's Therapy Centre: 'A woman's sense of self is formed in terms of and through her connection to others . . . loss of another person is likely to be experienced not as simply very sad, but as a terrifying loss of part of a woman's self or function in the world . . . any kind of loss can stimulate the feelings so many women have of not having been adequately loved as girls, their needs disallowed, their status inferior to that of boys. And the loss not of a person but of a job may exacerbate the already tenuous hold a woman feels she has on the outside world, her doubts about her rights and abilities to function outside the domestic sphere.'

According to this view depression isn't so much an illness as a result of things going wrong in our lives or relationships.

A psychologist who has carried out research into some of the reasons why people get depressed writes in the journal *New Scientist*: 'The reason that more women than men, and more people of lower socio-economic status . . . become depressed is quite simply that women and working-class people on average have lives with more possibility of things going seriously wrong, and fewer social and economic possibilities for dealing with the kinds of things that do go wrong.'

It's difficult to tease out distinct differences between anxiety and depression, since both tend to be two sides of the same coin. You may experience more symptoms connected with one than the other, but both may well be present. Psychologists have sometimes argued that depression is more concerned with our feelings about the past, while anxiety is to do with fears for the future, which when you think about it, seems to make a lot of sense.

Are you at risk of depression?

Research shows that some of us are more at risk of getting seriously depressed than others.

☐ Those with no paid work outside the home.

☐ Those with pre-school children.

☐ Those with three or more children under 14 living at home.

☐ Those on a low income.

☐ Those without the support of an intimate relationship.

☐ Those who have suffered a loss or bereavement early in life (especially if you have lost your mother before the age of eleven).

What sparks off depression?

Depression can be triggered off by many things including:

● Genetic factors.

● Life events (for a list of these see the Holmes-Rahe scale in the section on stress).

● Psychological factors. Some psychologists attribute depression to 'learned helplessness', when we feel so out of control of our lives and it seems pointless to even try. Others attribute depression to 'faulty thinking' i.e. the way we view the world affects our moods. Psychoanalytical theories see depression as being a result of aggression being turned inwards upon ourselves.

● Biochemical imbalances. For instance, an essential amino acid, Tryptophan has been found to be low in those suffering from depression.

● Environmental pollution and allergies.

● Low blood sugar.

● Drugs, including 'social' ones like alcohol, the Pill.

● Illnesses such as a bout of 'flu, glandular fever and so on.

● Accident or injury.

● Surgery e.g. mastectomy, hysterectomy.

● Fatigue and overwork.

● Menstrual problems.

● Loss of a job through retirement, redundancy or whatever.

● Divorce and separation or bereavement and the ensuing loneliness.

When to seek help

The point at which a depressed or anxious mood, which all of us suffer from time to time, tips over into 'illness' is a moot one, but if you've been experiencing any of the following for longer than a couple of weeks consider going to see your doctor or an alternative practitioner:

☐ You have no appetite and may have lost weight

☐ You feel constantly tired and all your get-up-and-go got up and went

☐ You can't get to sleep at night or you wake up early in the morning

☐ You feel agitated and on edge much of the time

☐ You can't summon any interest in things you used to enjoy

☐ You feel guilty and blame yourself for things that go wrong

☐ You have difficulty concentrating and are more indecisive than usual

☐ You've had thoughts of ending it all.

Orthodox treatment

When it comes to mental disorders there are signs that the conventional medical world is beginning to take social explanations more seriously. A recent article in the medical journal *The Practitioner* states: 'Patients with minor depression, vulnerable personalities or immediate life stresses can be helped by careful analysis of the problem, discussion and counselling.' Nevertheless, treatment with anti-depressants and tranquillizers is still the first line for more long-standing episodes of depression, the idea being that these can correct biochemical disturbances in the brain that are present in depression.

Anti-depressant drugs come in two types — the tricyclics which are used for moderate to severe depression, and the mono-amine oxidase inhibitors (MAOIs) which are prescribed if these haven't worked. The main problems with these drugs are that they don't *cure* depression. They work by acting on biochemical changes in your brain that are present in depression with the result that your sensitivity to emotions is reduced. What's more, they don't work for one out of three people.

And they take up to four weeks before they start to take effect. In the meantime, there may be several unpleasant side-effects including drowsiness, dry mouth, sight difficulties, nausea, constipation, shaking, rashes, sweating, sex and bladder problems, to mention a few. The MAOIs react with certain foods containing tyramine such as cheese, broad beans, meat or yeast extracts and certain red wines and sherry. That's not to say that these drugs can't provide a useful crutch for some of us to enable us to get over a difficult patch. But in the long run, masking the symptoms of depression can't cure broken nights, a crying baby, insufficient money to live on, or an unsatisfactory relationship with your partner. They can even, by encouraging you to define your problems as an 'illness', prevent you from trying to change things for the better or coming to terms with them.

If your doctor does prescribe a drug, make sure you know exactly what it is, why it's being prescribed, what side-effects you can

expect, how long you will have to take it, and how to come off. Some of the effects of coming off anti-depressants can be extremely severe and frightening, especially if you are not expecting them and if you have been on the drugs for a long time.

Tranquillizers

● One in five women take tranquillizers or sleeping pills at some time in the course of each year.

● Middle-aged women and those over 75 are most likely to be on tranquillizers.

● Tranquillizer use is higher if you don't have work outside the home.

Tranquillizers are frequently prescribed for anxiety, and if you have difficulty sleeping at night. The trouble is, tranquillizers are often being prescribed for the effects of much wider problems such as poor housing, lack of money, loneliness and so on. As one expert on tranquillizer use has put it: 'When the G.P. prescribes transquillizers he's putting *you* out of *his* misery.'

Tranquillizers can certainly be effective in the short term. But research shows that as time goes on they lose their efficiency. Even more seriously, if you've been on tranquillizers for a long time and then try to come off them suddenly you may experience a whole range of unpleasant and frightening withdrawal symptoms. And, as with anti-depressants they can stop you tackling the real problems that lie behind the symptoms of anxiety.

There simply isn't space in a book of this sort to go into detail into the question of tranquillizers. MIND, the National Association for Mental Health, list the following questions you should **ask your**

doctor if he prescribes tranquillizers:

1. *WHAT AND HOW?*

● What kind of tablets are they?

● How can they help me?

● How should they be taken?

● How can I see if they work?

2. *HOW IMPORTANT?*

● How important is it that I take them?

● What may happen if I do not take them?

3. *WHAT SIDE-EFFECTS?*

● Do they ever cause trouble?

● Do they have any side-effects?

● Can I drive after taking them?

● Can I take other medicines with them?

● Can I take alcohol when I am taking them?

4. *HOW LONG?*

● How long must I continue with these tablets?

● What should I do with tablets I do not need?

● Will I need to see you again?

● What will you want to know when I see you again?

Coming off tranquillizers

● Take it slowly. It's better to cut down gradually than to try to do it all at once.

● See a nutritional therapist or ask your doctor to recommend a vitamin and mineral supplement.

● Pay attention to your diet.

● Find out if there is a local support group in your area (contact your health visitor, G.P., local health education department, or MIND).

● Give yourself time.

● Be realistic. Don't expect it to be easy and don't punish yourself if you slip up from time to time.

● Relaxation, massage, visualization can all help.

● Get other people on your side so that they know how you are feeling and any difficulties you are having.

● Acupuncture may help you give up your addiction — but only if you really want to in the first place.

● If you feel the urge to take a pill, distract yourself, phone a friend, go for a walk, do some exercise, yoga or meditation.

● Try herbal treatment.

This is just the barest outline of a complex subject.

For further information:
Bottling it up, Valeri Curran and Susan Golombok, (Faber and Faber).

Coming off Tranquillizers: a withdrawal plan that really works, Shirley Trickett, (Thorsons).

Tranx, 17 Peel Road, Harrow, Middlesex HA3 7QX.

Mind, 22 Harley Street, London W1. (The special report *The price of tranquillity* is especially detailed and useful.)

Trouble with Tranquillizers published by Release, 1-4 Hatton Gardens, London EC1N 8ND.

Alternative approaches to mental health

Given the side effects and other problems of orthodox treatments for mental problems, what does alternative medicine have to offer?

The area is one in which almost any of the alternative therapies can prove useful, even some that on the surface may seem unpromising such as acupuncture. A woman acupuncturist quoted in *Dealing with Depression* by Kathy Nairne and Gerrilyn Smith, Women's Press, says: 'The needles by themselves can do much to calm agitated energy or to raise it in cases of physical or mental depletion. There are specific treatments which in some cases can re-establish balance almost miraculously in people who are seriously disturbed . . . However in many cases a rearrangement of lifestyle is necessary if the treatment is to be effective.'

The final sentence is perhaps an explanation of why the alternative therapies can be so helpful. Following the guidelines laid out in part one of the book can provide a useful basis.

As always, *diet* plays a large part in the alternative approach. Professor Bryce-Smith of Reading has written on the role zinc deficiency may play in depression. As pointed out in the chapter on premenstrual syndrome vitamin B_6 can also be useful. The Pill is known to leach the body of B_6 which may explain why some women using it suffer depression. The amino acid tryptophan has been found to be low in people suffering depression. Taking supplements of this seems to result in improvements that can be usefully compared to standard anti-depressant drugs. This is one 'alternative' therapy you may be able to get from an orthodox doctor. You shouldn't take it if you are on MAOI anti-depressants as it can cause eyesight problems and headaches, nor should you take it if you are suffering from bladder disease.

Homoeopathy has a wide number of remedies, which as always, are linked to particular personality types.

On the *herbal* side, infusions such as lemon balm, oats, vervain or camomile are helpful in mild cases. More powerful herbal remedies can be very useful, and you should consult a qualified herbalist.

Most of the *mind-body* therapies such as Yoga, Meditation, Alexander Technique and relaxation programmes can help, as can various types of psychotherapeutic techniques outlined in the last part of the book.

PART THREE

Fertility and Reproduction

Contraception

Like it or not, most women's lives are bound up with their fertility. The whole question of reproduction is one that has been medicalized to the nth degree. Better family planning methods have been responsible for women's greater longevity — very few of us die in childbirth nowadays; for smaller families; and for the fact that women today can be more independent than their grandmothers. On the face of it there is more choice than ever before in contraception. Yet some of us — and it is overwhelmingly women who take responsibility for contraceptive measures — find it difficult to choose what is the best sort for us.

All present contraceptive methods have their drawbacks, and the type of contraception you need will depend to a large extent on your age and the stage of life you are at. For instance, if you don't have a regular sex life, it's pretty pointless to be on the Pill. If you just want contraception to space children, rather than because you have finished your family, your priorities in choosing a method will be different. The whole issue is even more complicated because the Pill, which at one time seemed about to herald a new age of freedom, has come under ever-growing clouds of

suspicion on health grounds. This section looks at orthodox contraceptive methods, and then looks at how viable natural family planning methods are as an alternative.

Orthodox contraceptive methods

Method
Barrier methods e.g. cap, sheath.

Effectiveness
Varies between 85 and 99 per cent depending on how carefully you use them.

Safety
Extremely safe, though some women are allergic to rubber or spermicides. Sheath offers some protection against sexually transmitted diseases and cervical cancer. Cystitis sometimes a problem with some types of diaphragm.

Advantages
Flexible, especially if you aren't in a regular sexual partnership. Can be used long or short term. Helps you to get used to handling your own body and to feel at ease with it.

Disadvantages
May interfere with spontaneity. Some couples dislike using a spermicide and find

Diaphragm in place

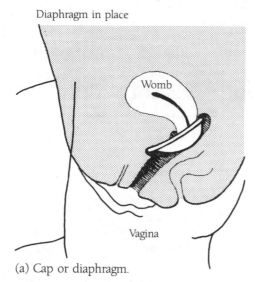

(a) Cap or diaphragm.

(b) Sheath.

Figure 11:

it messy and unaesthetic. Some men complain sheath reduces sensation during lovemaking. May be implicated in vaginal infections.

Method
The Pill.

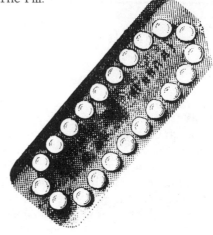

Figure 12: The Pill.

Effectiveness
Very effective. The combined pill is 99-99.9 per cent effective. The mini-pill (progestogen only) 96-98 per cent.

Safety
An increasing body of evidence points to quite considerable disadvantages. Some recent studies appear to point to a connection between long term use of the Pill and breast cancer. But others dismiss such suggestions. However, the Pill seems to offer some protection against ovarian cancer, cancer of the body of the uterus, some pelvic infections, and rheumatoid arthritis.

Advantages

Extremely effective if you definitely don't want to become pregnant. Its action is continuous so you can have sex any time without the fear of getting pregnant. It doesn't interrupt lovemaking.

Disadvantages

Reduced effectiveness if you have had a bout of diarrhoea, forget to take it, or are on certain drugs e.g. antibiotics. Side-effects range from those which are a nuisance — such as weight gain, depression, loss of sexual desire — to high blood-pressure, migraine, gall-bladder disease. Possible cancer risk as already outlined. Associated with higher rate of cervical erosion. Depletes the body of several important nutrients e.g. vitamin C, zinc. Sometimes makes PMS worse.

You should avoid taking a high-dose Pill if any of the following apply:

- [ ] You are pregnant
- [ ] You have a history of thrombosis
- [ ] You have had cancer of the breast or genitals
- [ ] You smoke
- [ ] You get migraine
- [ ] You have existing high blood-pressure
- [ ] You are diabetic
- [ ] You are overweight
- [ ] You have severe varicose veins
- [ ] You are over thirty-five
- [ ] There's a family history of thrombosis or hyperlipidaemia (i.e. a high level of fats in the blood).

Methods

Intra-uterine contraceptive device (IUCD or IUD).

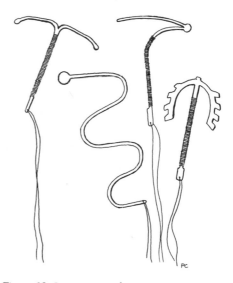

Figure 13: Intrauterine devices (IUD).

Effectiveness

About 97 per cent if you have already had children, slightly less good if you haven't.

Advantages

Once in place you can forget about it, only needing replacing every two to five years, depending on type.

Disadvantages

Can make your periods heavier and more painful. Increased risk of pelvic inflammatory disease (PID), particularly if you are younger and have more than one sexual partner, which can impair future fertility. If you get pregnant while using an IUD, there is an increased risk of ectopic pregnancy or miscarriage. In rare instances may perforate uterus. May drop out without you noticing.

Method

Depo-Provera or Noristerat. A form of progestogen is given as a long-lasting injection which lasts for 2 to 3 months.

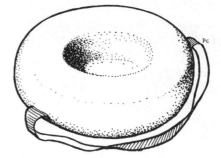

Figure 15: Collatex sponge.

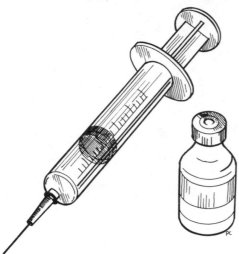

Figure 14: Injectable contraception.

Effectiveness
Extremely effective — over 99 per cent.

Advantages
Once it's been done you can forget about it.

Disadvantages
Can't be stopped if you change your mind. Drug stays in your body 8 to 10 months. Can cause either heavy, irregular bleeding or stop periods altogether. Side-effects include weight gain, headache, depression, backache, reduced sexual desire, nausea, abdominal discomfort, acne. May take up to 2 years before fertility returns.

Method
Collatex sponge — contains spermicide.

Effectiveness
From 75-91 per cent as far as is known so far. Thought to be less effective in women who have had children and whose vaginas have been stretched.

Advantages
May be more comfortable and less messy than cap. Repeated intercourse can occur without the need for extra spermicide. No fitting required — one size fits all.

Disadvantages
As for other barrier methods. But, unlike cap, sponge should not be used during a period. Not widely available on the NHS.

Method
Morning-after Pill (post-coital contraception). A special high dose Pill is used within 3 days of unprotected intercourse (2 tablets followed by another 2 twelve hours later).

Effectiveness
Said to be 99 per cent effective.

Safety
If the method fails hormones could affect baby.

Advantages
Avoids having to have abortion if it is important you have not become pregnant.

Disadvantages
Nausea and vomiting. Withdrawal bleeding. Only to be used in extreme emergency.

Method
Post-coital IUD. Another morning-after method which is effective up to five days after unprotected intercourse.

Effectiveness
100 per cent effective so far as we know.

Advantages
Can be used as on-going method, if wished.

Disadvantages
As for IUD.

Method
Sterilization — either vasectomy for man or tubal litigation (when Fallopian tubes are clipped, tied or cut) for woman.

Effectiveness
Virtually 100 per cent.

Disadvantages
Some women experience heavier, more painful periods or irregular bleeding. You can't change your mind.

Further information:
Family Planning Information Service, 27-35 Mortimer Street, London W1N 7RJ. Tel: 01-636 7866. Write or 'phone for advice or leaflets.

Alternative methods of family planning
The risks and drawbacks already outlined of conventional family planning methods have led many to explore natural family planning methods. It's important to distinguish between the new natural techniques and the old-fashioned 'rhythm' method, which well earned the tag 'Vatican roulette' because of its high failure rate.

The new techniques are neither haphazard nor unscientific — they are based on careful and accurate observation of the signs and symptoms of fertility. However, they do demand a degree of dedication and self discipline that some women find irksome.

How does it work?
Natural family planning techniques make use of the fact that you can only conceive during about three to six days each month. In fact, over your whole lifetime you are fertile for a mere 4 per cent of the time. Given the relatively restricted time during which conception can occur, natural family planning experts argue that taking precautions every single time you make love is using a sledgehammer to crack a nut.

Natural family planning methods based on careful observation of the fertile period are, *when used properly*, claimed to be as effective as the Pill in preventing an unwanted pregnancy. The biggest bonus of course is that they are entirely free of side-effects.

Fertility awareness
The key to natural family planning is fertility awareness. That means having a basic knowledge of the way in which your body prepares itself for pregnancy each month, plus an understanding of your partner's potential fertility.

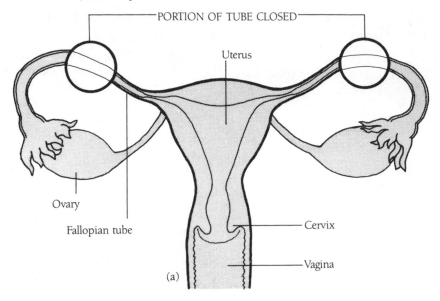

(a)

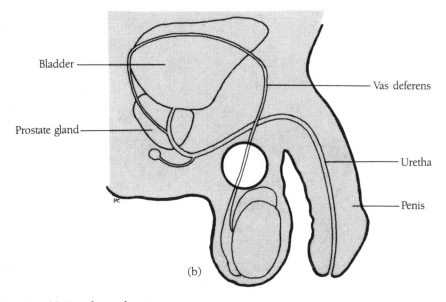

(b)

Figure 16: (a) Female sterilization.
         (b) Male sterilization.

Once the ovum is released it has a lifespan of 12 to 36 hours. If it is not fertilized by the sperm during this time it dies and is shed during your period. Your partner on the other hand can be 100 per cent fertile from puberty onwards. The life of a sperm can be anything from a few hours to up to 4 days during which it can fertilize the egg if conditions are favourable. Add the two together and that makes about 6 days altogether when you *could* get pregnant.

Whether a sperm survives and makes it to the egg depends on the mucus produced by your cervix under the influence of oestrogen and progesterone. Immediately after your period, oestrogen levels are low and the mucus produced by the cervix is thick, but there isn't much of it. It literally blocks the sperms and prevents it from entering the uterus. As ovulation gets nearer, oestrogen levels rise and the mucus produced becomes clear, slippery and favourable to sperm: it both nourishes the sperm and creates 'tracks' along which it can move rapidly towards the uterus. Oestrogen levels peak about 40 hours before the egg is released and then fall.

A few days after ovulation progesterone takes over. The mucus again becomes hostile to sperm and conception cannot occur. The potential fertility of you and your partner therefore depends on the lifespan of the egg combined with the lifespan of the sperm. Natural family planning means you can work with the natural cycle, either abstaining from sex or using a barrier method during the short period when conception can occur.

There are two main methods of natural birth control: the mucus method and the sympto-thermal method.

The mucus method

This is also known as the ovulation or Billings method and relies on the observation of mucus changes already outlined. It is basically a method of predicting ovulation before it happens. The first day of a period is counted as day one, and since it is virtually impossible to detect mucus during menstruation, this is considered a potentially fertile time. After a period most women experience a 'dry' spell when the mucus produced is scanty, thick, opaque and hostile to sperm. The fertile phase begins when wet, thin, stringy mucus begins to be produced. You can detect the mucus either by wiping your vaginal entrance with a tissue before going to the toilet, or by inserting a finger and taking a sample from the cervix. As ovulation approaches the mucus becomes increasingly favourable to sperm. It is wet and lubricative and can be stretched between thumb and forefinger like raw egg white. Ovulation usually occurs within two days of the appearance of this type of mucus. After that it becomes thick, sticky, and clotty or disappears altogether.

All in all you are potentially fertile during your period and during the 'wet' days plus an extra four days to allow for the lifespan of the egg and the possibility of a second ovulation (when this occurs it's always within a few hours of the first). The last days of the cycle, about 10 days in all, are infertile. The phase of the cycle leading up to ovulation can vary a lot from woman to woman and from month to month, and it is this variation which is responsible for the different lengths of cycle we all experience. The second phase of the cycle — from ovulation to menstruation is around 14 days.

Observation of mucus can be especially useful if you are breast-feeding and have not yet restarted your periods, as it can tell you whether you are ovulating, which is useful if you don't want to get pregnant again soon. Fertility usually returns gradually as the baby has fewer breast-feeds and this may be marked by 'patchy' mucus, indicating that the body is trying to ovulate.

The sympto-thermal methods

This combines these mucus observations with recordings of the temperature changes which determine the safe time *after* ovulation. In addition you are encouraged to notice other cyclical changes such as breast tenderness, alternations in the position of the cervix, mood changes and so on. In this way it is possible to pin down the fertile period with some accuracy.

The basis of the sympto-thermal method is temperature recording. The lining of the uterus has been compared to an incubator which every month gets warm ready to receive a baby, under the influence of progesterone. The resting temperature of the body (Basal Body Temperature or BBT) is recorded at the same time every day. During the early part of the cycle, under the influence of oestrogen, the BBT remains low. After ovulation the presence of progesterone in the bloodstream causes a slight rise in BBT. If you don't become pregnant your temperature will drop again either just before or during your period. If you do conceive the high level of circulating progesterone which continues for the first three months of pregnancy means that your temperature will remain high. For this reason changes in temperature can be used as an indicator of pregnancy long before either chemical tests or physical examination would show up as positive.

The rise in temperature is only slight (about 0.2 to 0.5°C, 0.4 to 0.6°F) so it is a good idea to use a specially calibrated 'fertility' thermometer (available from large chemists or the Family Planning Association) rather than the ordinary fever kind, which is more difficult to read.

A good time to take your temperature is first thing in the morning *before* getting up. You can take it by mouth, vaginally or rectally. Since an ovum lives for 12 to 36 hours, you should avoid unprotected intercourse for two whole days of higher temperature. In other words you need to have recorded *three* higher temperatures. Women who use the method say taking daily temperature readings becomes such a habit that it is no more bother than cleaning your teeth or brushing your hair.

In addition to temperature and mucus observations you may notice other signs of ovulation. Many women experience pain or a small amount of mid-cycle bleeding when they ovulate. Another good indicator is the position of the cervix. During the early part of the cycle the cervix is low and you can touch it with your finger. The opening, or os, is closed. Towards ovulation the cervix is pulled higher into the vagina by the ligaments which support it, and the os opens slightly, especially if you have had children. Other signs of the later part of the cycle include such premenstrual symptoms as bloating, weight gain, breast tenderness and emotional changes.

Special circumstances

If you've just had a baby it can be difficult to observe fertility signs, especially if you are up several times a night, and generally run off your feet. As soon as the lochia (the discharge after the childbirth) has stopped you can start observing mucus again. If you are breastfeeding completely on demand and frequently, you are unlikely to be fertile, but keep up your observations so that returning fertility doesn't catch you unawares.

Vaginal infection
A vaginal infection will make observation of mucus difficult, especially if you are using any creams, pessaries or ointments to treat it. You can continue to take your temperature and start checking mucus again as soon as you are sure the infection has completely healed.

Premenstrual syndrome
Because of hormone imbalances that may occur as part of PMS your mucus patterns may be somewhat irregular. Treating your PMS according to the guidelines laid down earlier may make fertility signs easier to identify. Since PMS symptoms are often made worse by the Pill and IUD, natural family planning methods may be especially suitable if you are a sufferer.

Further advice on dealing with special circumstances is available in the books listed at the end of this section. Of course the big question is 'Does it work?' Dr Anna Flynn a leading expert on natural family planning says, 'As with all types of contraception the success or failure of the methods depends on how much the couple want to avoid pregnancy. For example, in one Canadian survey the method was 99 per cent effective for women who had finished their families, as opposed to 93 per cent for those who were merely using it to space children.' These figures compare favourably with more established methods such as the Pill and IUD. The secret of success seems to be strong motivation and good teaching. A short chapter such as this can't do more than lay down the basic outlines of the method. For further detail either get hold of one of the books mentioned, or better still go to one of the natural family planning courses held by one of the organizations listed below.

There are two physical circumstances in which natural family planning techniques might be impracticable. The first is if you have a cervical erosion, since this produces its own mucus. The second where the cervix has been cauterized since after the initial treatment no mucus is produced.

There are various kits and gadgets on the market that can aid fertility awareness. However they are all a bit expensive, and despite new advances many are somewhat hit and miss. Most natural family planning experts would argue that though such gadgets may be useful they are no real substitute for knowing your own body's individual rhythms.

Lunaception
A method of contraception that determines ovulation by the moon. Moonlight is known to influence the menstrual cycle. An American, Louise Lacey, has discovered that it's possible to use light to regulate the cycle so as to make it a means of birth control. However there's no firm evidence as yet upon the efficacy of such methods.

Astrological birth control
Again based on the relationship of the sun and moon, the idea being that your fertile period is determined by the angles of the sun and moon in the sky at the time of your birth. For two days before this you are in your 'cosmic fertility period' and able to conceive. Nowadays it's usually combined with some sort of rhythm method. However it's only fair to say that the whole thing is a bit iffy, even though it's said to be widely used in Eastern Europe.

Further information:
A Manual of Natural Family Planning, Dr Anna Flynn, (Allen and Unwin).
Fertility Awareness Workbook, Barbara Kass-Annese & Dr Hal Danzer, (Thorsons).
Natural birth control, Katia and Jonathan Drake, (Thorsons).

To find a teacher in your area contact:
Natural Family Planning Unit, Birmingham Maternity Unit, Queen Elizabeth Medical Centre, Birmingham B15 2TG.

Katia and Jonathan Drake, 12 Priestley House, Athlone Street, London NW5 4LP.

Natural Family Planning Service, Catholic Marriage Advisory Council, 15 Lansdowne Road, London W11 3AJ.

Infertility

About one in six couples has difficulty conceiving. In fact the term 'infertile' is perhaps inaccurate, since in many cases the problem turns out to be 'subfertility'. In other words they are able to conceive but for one reason or another, for instance sexual difficulties, stress or malnutrition, the system needs a bit of a kick to get it into action.

Infertility problems have increased in recent years — the reasons for this increase include the fact that more of us are putting off having a family until over age 30 when fertility is starting to decline, and secondly the increase in sexually transmitted diseases (outlined earlier in the book).

The whole field is an area where orthodox and alternative cross each other. Many orthodox practitioners would agree that modern drugs and environmental chemicals play a part in reducing fertility, either because they affect the absorption of nutrients from the diet which are necessary for a healthy hormone balance (for instance too much cadmium may result in zinc deficiency which has been linked to male infertility), or because they affect the sperm directly.

What are the main causes of infertility?

For women:

● *Damaged Fallopian tubes, ovaries or uterus.* This usually results from a previous infection inside or outside the tubes (PID), following a ruptured appendix, or pelvic abcess or from complications following a miscarriage, abortion or difficult birth. More rarely the tubes have been malformed from birth. Signs that your tubes may be damaged are pain during intercourse, general pelvic aching and irregular periods.

● *Endometriosis* (see vaginal infections for further details). This is when tissue that normally lines the womb implants in other parts of the body. The main symptoms are pain during intercourse, heavy and painful bleeding.

● *Hormone imblances* resulting in failure to ovulate or irregular ovulation. Possible, symptoms are short, irregular or absent periods.

● *Problems affecting the cervix and uterus.* Cervical infection or erosion can cause subfertility. Some cervical mucus is 'hostile' to sperm preventing it from passing into the uterus. Fibroids can also affect the ability to conceive.

● *Being very overweight or underweight,* which affects the hormone balance.

For men:

● *Low sperm count or no sperm.* This may have been caused by mumps; the effects of certain drugs; surgical damage — for instance from a hernia operation; the sperms being stored at too high a temperature through undescended testicle, overweight or even tight jeans and trousers, sexually transmitted diseases; hormonal imbalance; overweight; just as women are sometimes allergic to their partner's sperm, men too sometimes form antibodies against their own sperm; finally making love too often can lower the sperm count.

● *Poor quality sperm* this can result from hormonal imbalance; varicocele — a sort of varicose vein of the testes; or hydrocele — a bag of fluid in the scrotum, inflammation of the prostate gland; or too much or too little semen.

● *Blocked tubes* caused by scarring from infection or sexually transmitted disease or where the tubes are twisted.

Other factors

These include various medical conditions such as TB or other severe illnesses; disorders of the endocrine system, like diabetes; infections of the genital or urinary systems such as thrush or cystitis. Then there are the sexual problems of a physical or emotional origin — for instance in the man the failure to achieve or maintain an erection, in the woman a vagina that is too tight or goes into spasm during intercourse. Even something as simple as sexual technique can be to blame for some problems. The sperm needs to be deposited high in the vagina if it is to stand the best chance of entering the cervix and fertilizing an egg. Sexual positions where the penis can penetrate deeply are best. For conception to occur ideally the semen should bathe the cervix for at least half an hour after intercourse, so obviously if you leap up and wash yourself immediately after making love you aren't really giving nature a fair chance. This may present you with a problem if for example you suffer from cystitis, which is why it's worth getting such problems cleared up before trying to conceive.

What treatment is available?

A full medical history and examination will be carried out on both of you. The whole business may be rather depressing, and you could well be letting yourself in for a whole series of tests and investigations spanning several years. There may be long waits between appointments. Despite the large numbers of infertile couples infertility services are woefully inadequate.

Investigations

● **Semen analysis or sperm count.** The first and most basic test carried out on the man. It involves your partner masturbating into a clean container. The sperm will be tested for their mobility and shape to make sure they are normal. Usually this will be done several times over a period of months.

● **Post-coital test.** Cervical mucus is examined after intercourse to see how receptive it is to the sperm, whether it is hostile or too thick.

● **Further male tests.** These include measurements of gonadotrophin levels and tests to see whether your partner is infertile for genetic reasons.

● **Ovulation tests.** These include several of the techniques already outlined in natural family planning i.e.
  i. taking your temperature daily
  ii. cervical mucus test
  iii. measurement of hormone levels

● **Endometrial biopsy.** A scraping of tissue is taken from the lining of your uterus to see if ovulation has taken place.

● **Laparoscopy.** A complex test which enables the doctor to look at your ovaries. Fallopian tubes and uterus. The abdomen is blown up with carbon dioxide so that space exists between your pelvic organs. Then an instrument like a telescope (laparoscope) is passed through a small cut near your navel. This enables the surgeon to check for fibroids, endometriosis and blocked Fallopian tubes.

● **Hysterosalpingogram.** This test shows the position of any obstruction in the tubes and the internal structure of the uterus, by means of a water-soluble dye which is injected into the cervix. A series of X-ray pictures which will show the site of any blockage is then taken.

Orthodox treatment

The sort of treatment you will need depends on your medical history and the results of the various tests. Sometimes all that is necessary is to clear up local infection, or simple advice on timing of intercourse. Simple self-help techniques like douching the vagina to make it more alkaline (for example with bicarb) or acid (see vaginal infections) can make the environment more favourable to sperm. Men can be helped by simple advice to wear loose fitting underpants and avoiding tight jeans or trousers; bathing the testes in cold water every day; cutting down on alcohol or going on a diet. Often simple measures such as these do the trick.

Where these don't work there are two main lines of treatment — hormonal and surgical. Both of these have progressed by leaps and bounds during the last few years. The commonest 'fertility drug' is Clomid, which is taken daily from the second to fifth days of your cycle to stimulate ovulation. Pergonal is a gonadotrophin (a hormone released by the pituitary) which is given by injection. It's the drug that tends to stimulate multiple pregnancy if not given in a very carefully controlled dose. Newer techniques involve 'hormone releasing factors', which control ovulation, administered by means of a small portable pump, about the size of a cigarette packet, that is strapped to your arm or leg.

Hormone treatment for men is less successful, though oddly enough, some men have been successfully treated using human chorionic gonadotrophins of the sort used to stimulate ovulation in women. And there is hope that hormone releasing factors may be of use to men too.

Surgery involves operations to remove fibroids or cysts if they are interfering with conception, or to correct any abnormalities of the reproductive system. Some of the most dramatic advances recently are in the area of tubal microsurgery that seems to offer a better chance of unblocking tubes, reshaping the entrance to the tube and removing scar tissue (adhesions) than more conventional techniques.

Other methods of treating infertility include test tube fertilization (IVF) in which embryos fertilized outside the woman's body are replaced at the entrance of the uterus by means of a fine tube and artificial insemination (either by husband or by an anonymous donor — AIH and AID respectively).

Alternative approaches

Despite the successes of modern medicine in treating infertility, a small number of couples find themselves unable to conceive, for no very good reason. This can be where alternative techniques come in.

Stress

Stress seems to play a major part in many cases of unexplained infertility — hence the common experience of couples who conceive immediately after they have started adoption proceedings. A *relaxation and exercise programme* as outlined in part one of the book can certainly help. *Hypnosis* has recently been shown to be effective in some women experiencing repeated miscarriage. The stress that undergoing treatment can have on a relationship shouldn't be ignored either. One couple make the following point in an article in *Mother and Baby* magazine October 1984: 'Infertility is an enormous strain on a relationship. At first it's easy to laugh at having to have intercourse to order, but that palls after a while and you begin to feel a freak. Talking to other people and realizing there are others in the same boat eases the pain.'

Joining a support group such as CHILD or NAC can help.

Meditation and yoga can be useful too.

Eating a good wholefood diet, cutting out coffee and tea and smoking. One study in the *BMJ* June 8th 1985 showed that even as few as ten cigarettes a day can reduce fertility.

Supplements

Some experts advise supplementation with *vitamin C* and amino acids such as arginine for low sperm count, while amino acid *cartinine* found in avocado pear is said to affect sperm motility. *Zinc* has been found to be low in some couples suffering from infertility. But a word of warning: too much zinc can suppress your immune system according to a report in the *Journal of Alternative Medicine* August 1986. As always you should only take supplements under the supervision of a nutritional practitioner.

Cold hip baths may aid poor sperm production.

Homoeopathy/herbalism

Where infertility is associated with adhesions in the internal organs a homoeopathic/herbal approach is sometimes successful. An alternative practitioner who is also medically qualified

warns that couples shouldn't pin all their hopes on such methods. 'If they are going to work they will usually have done so by three to six months of treatment', he says.

Hormone problems can be treated by a clinical ecology approach, in which homoeopathic dosages of progesterone and oestrogen are given. The herb *agnus vitex castus* Chaste-berry, is especially useful for helping rebalance hormone levels where this is a problem. A medical herbalist comments that herbal treatment can be very successful in cases of hostile mucus.

Acupuncture

Ear acupuncture (auricular) can often make a significant contribution where the menstrual cycle is irregular. One South African gynaecologist in a small scale study of 15 to 20 patients found that 60 per cent got preg-

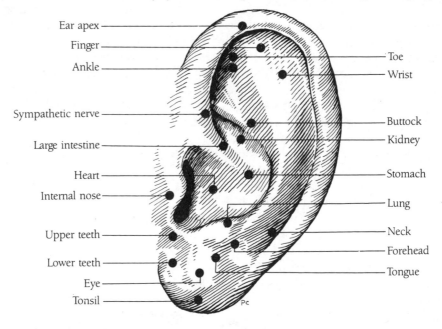

Figure 17: Ear acupuncture points.

nant within three months using this method.

The practitioner I mentioned earlier warns: 'Infertility is an extremely complex subject and requires someone who understands both complementary and orthodox methods. Unfortunately, these are few and far between.' When should you give up? This practitioner says: 'It's a difficult question and there are no clear rules, a lot depends on age. I'm very much against people being conned when there is no hope. I'd say after 6 to 9 months of treatment you should think carefully about whether or not to continue.'

Finally, before leaving the subject of infertility, here are some anecdotal reports culled from the pages of the NAC newsletter: 'I overcame my fertility problems, investigated but not conclusive, with acupuncture. In early pregnancy I was taught self-hypnosis and have to date had three sessions. I have found it to be of tremendous help in that it has given me confidence.'

Another writer describing long-standing problems with ovarian cysts and blocked Fallopian tubes says: 'I began acupuncture treatments, thinking it might help me to relax if nothing else. I also took Clomiphere for one cycle. One month later I was pregnant! It would seem to be a combination of factors which did the trick. A sympathetic, caring

consultant and the encouragement of a skilled acupuncturist, advice on diet and stress (I previously drank up to six cups of coffee daily) and just the knowledge that my perseverance and decisive action was getting me somewhere — all played their part.'

She adds: 'You must not give up until you have explored areas such as acupuncture and homoeopathy. These treatments can be complementary to whatever medical treatment is being received.'

Finally, a carroty tale: 'After three years of infertility tests, no treatment and no joy, we had given up any hope of having a baby. My husband had a very low sperm count and poor motility . . . I read about the carrot diet. and decided to feed my husband on carrots with most meals. This was last May. In July I was pregnant. Whether the carrots had anything to do with our success we shall never know. But to any couples with the same problem as ours, I would say it is worth a try.'

Further information:
Infertility — A Common-Sense Guide for the Childless, Andrew Stanway, (Thorsons).

National Association for the Childless (NAC) 318 Summer Lane, Birmingham B19 3RL.

CHILD Farthings, Gaunts Road, Pawlett, Nr Bridgwater, Somerset.

Pre-conceptional care

The idea of encouraging women and men to lead a healthy life before pregnancy has hit the headlines in the last few years. There's a fair body of evidence to suggest that getting fit and well before conception can help avoid some problems later in pregnancy. The incidence of spina bifida and similar defects

for instance has been shown in trials to be reduced in women taking a vitamin and mineral supplement before pregnancy. And certainly no one would argue with the advice to avoid non-essential prescription and over-the-counter drugs. But a large number of alternative practitioners go one step further.

Far too many women, they argue, enter pregnancy mildly malnourished. The Pill disturbs the metabolism and alters the balance of nutrients in the body. They may have been living on a diet of convenience foods and restaurant meals. And they may be suffering from allergies or minor infections such as cystitis or thrush, which can impair the body's ability to absorb food or deplete it of certain nutrients.

In addition, some women are overweight or have been dieting. Add on the well-publicized dangers of smoking, drinking and environmental pollutants all of which are known, — at least to some extent to cross the placenta — and, claim these experts, you have potential for disaster. 'A woman may be healthy enough for all normal purposes but when it comes to taking on the additional burden of pregnancy and feeding another human being it may be different,' says a clinical ecologist, working in the field.

The organization Foresight was formed by parents, backed by doctors and nutritionists, to publicize the need for care before pregnancy begins — preconceptional care. In its 40 private clinics, couples can — for a price — undergo a thorough medical overhaul with the option of special tests such as hair analysis to show the presence of toxic minerals in the body or a lack of essential ones. It's mainly over this question that the Foresight brigade are at odds with the orthodox medics. It's not that orthodox doctors dismiss preconceptional care, indeed in a few areas pre-pregnancy clinics are held under the auspices of the NHS. But hair analysis as a diagnostic technique has come in for a lot of stick. Dr Barbara Pickard, who is by no means unsympathetic to the idea of pre-pregnancy care, sums up the situation well in her book *Eating Well for a*

Healthy Pregnancy (Sheldon): 'The technique is worthless for vitamins and the problems of mineral analysis centre on the overwhelming difficulties involved in the interpretation of hair-charts. Many things can affect the levels of minerals in the hair — the external environment, washing procedures, hair treatments such as dyes, perms and even shampoos which contain minerals such as selenium or zinc, the natural colour of hair, the person's age and sex, the season of the year and the rate of hair growth. The levels of minerals in the hair do not often correspond to the levels in blood, urine or saliva which makes it even more difficult to relate the values to your own health. One area in which hair analysis *may* prove useful is in the detection of high levels of toxic minerals such as lead, mercury and cadmium. A high result here would be well worth following up with further tests of blood and urine.'

Controversy also rages over the use of vitamin and mineral supplements for women who are not at risk of having a handicapped baby. It's a very similar argument to the one outlined in the chapter on diet. What's more, organizations such as the Spastics Society and the Maternity Alliance warn that preconceptional care as offered by Foresight, aimed as it is at well-heeled middle class couples who can afford the service, fails to reach those very women who would most benefit from it — teenage mothers and those who are alone, those on a low income, the unemployed and those living in poor housing. Such organizations would prefer to see preconceptional care being part of a much wider health education process extending into schools and family planning clinics.

There's also the effect that preconceptional

propaganda can have on the peace of mind of pregnant women. After all, most babies aren't handicapped, despite the fact that most of us don't go for pre-pregnancy care. As Faith Haddad, a London obstetrician, is quoted as saying in *Options* November, 1986: 'They're almost implying that if a woman has a miscarriage or abnormal baby then she must have done something wrong. It's awfully hard for a woman to carry that guilt. Nobody's perfect. I've had people ring me up to say they went to a party and had three glasses of wine and are worried that they might have been in the first stages of pregnancy at the time. It promotes anxiety.' As the article goes on to point out, anxiety in itself can lead to a more difficult labour.

So what should you make of it all? By all means try to get yourself fit and well before getting pregnant. But ordinary common-sense measures such as those given in part one will usually be sufficient to ensure that you are in good health. It's also sensible to make sure you haven't any lurking infections such as thrush or cystitis, and the alternative approaches described earlier can help here. As for vitamin and mineral supplements — as always you pays your money — and in some cases this can be quite considerable — and you takes your choice. If you've previously given birth to a handicapped baby, it may be worth consulting a practitioner interested in nutritional methods before getting pregnant in case he thinks a multi-vitamin and mineral supplement is advisable. However chances are that even if you don't do any of these things you'll have a perfectly healthy baby. And it could be argued that stress reduction is equally as important in the prevention of premature and low birth weight babies as any other sort of treatment. And in fact trials are now in progress at four maternity hospitals to look into the effect that lowering stress, through a tailor-made counselling programme, might have on birth weight.

Having a healthy pregnancy

The secret of having a healthy pregnancy is to pay special attention to the areas of your life outlined in part one. Eat a good wholefood diet, get enough exercise and relaxation and cut stress to the minimum. There are lots of new things going on in your life when you are pregnant, and a whole different set of circumstances to adjust to. The growth of a new life inside you may make you especially open to the spiritual side of life. Many women find meditation and guided fantasy work especially creative and uplifting when they are pregnant.

What should I eat?
By and large the rules for healthy eating are the same during pregnancy as at any other time. Concentrate on getting fresh, good quality foods, choosing a few foods from the following four food groups:
1. *Dairy products* — milk, yogurt, cheese.
2. *Proteins* — nuts, beans, seeds, meat, fish and eggs.
3. *Vegetables and fruit* — green leafy vegetables, dried fruits, any other fruit and vegetables in season, juices.
4. *Bread and cereals* — brown rice and other

whole grains, muesli, porridge, wholemeal bread, wholewheat or rye crispbread.

At one time there were strict limits placed on how much weight women were supposed to gain in pregnancy. Today this is much more flexible. Unless you are very overweight it's undesirable to diet when you are pregnant. If you do need to lose weight it's best to do it under supervision, so ask your midwife or a qualified practitioner interested in nutritional methods.

There's some evidence that if you are very underweight when you start pregnancy, you are more at risk of giving birth to a low birth weight baby. The answer is to use the stress relieving measures outlined in part one, and eat a good diet of the type described above and elsewhere.

As for eating for two, not many of us believe you have to do that nowadays. In fact if you did, you would probably end up vastly overweight. But a new study just carried out in Edinburgh and London suggests that the recommended level of 2,400 calories a day for pregnant women might be set too high. Women in the study whose average food intakes were 2,000 to 2,200 calories produced perfectly healthy babies and the premature birth rate was lower than expected.

Minor ailments of pregnancy

Pregnancy is not an illness. Even so, many women are plagued by a number of irritating minor ailments. It's best to avoid taking any drugs unless they are prescribed by your doctor during pregnancy, and this is where alternative remedies can be so helpful.

Morning sickness

About half of all women suffer some degree of nausea or vomiting in early pregnancy. It's thought to be due to increased levels of the hormone human chorionic gonadotrophin (HCG) which is produced early on in pregnancy. In very severe cases (hyperemesis) there may be a psychological component in which case any of the mind-body therapies may be especially useful, particularly if you want to avoid hospital admission.

Herbal remedies for morning sickness include camomile or peppermint tea. Ginger — either a quarter of an ounce of crystallized or grated root ginger added to a cup of boiling water with honey to taste, or a teaspoon of dried ginger, may be helpful too.

Homoeopathic remedies are also useful for morning sickness. The following, quoted in *Birth Matters*, edited by Ros Claxton, (Unwin Paperbacks), are especially useful:

Ipecacuanha — you feel irritable and resentful about the pregnancy.
Sepia — you feel indifferent towards those you love, depressed and can't stand noise and smells.
Phosphorus — indifferent but crave sympathy. You are anxious about others and afraid of being on your own. You crave fresh air and cold drinks, but may be sick after them.
Pulsatilla — you weep easily, are moody and crave sympathy.
Ignatia — you do unexpected irrational things.
Aurum — if you are deeply depressed. Self-help homoeopathic remedies are best taken in the 6th potency, if these aren't effective, see a qualified

homoeopath to see whether a more powerful potency is recommended.

Diet may also play a part in helping to avoid morning sickness. Eat, small, regular meals. These are some other tricks worth trying:

Rest — get regular rest periods during the day. See if you can arrange with your boss to go in a bit later to avoid the rush hour. Try to get one or two early nights a week. Avoid non-essential housework.

Diet — avoid highly spiced or fatty foods. Go for milky drinks and soup if you can't keep anything down. Drink spa waters and fruit juices rather than tea and coffee which can increase nausea. Keep a hoard of snacks to nibble on and off during the day.

Supplements — Vitamin B_6 seems to help some women. But don't overdo it — consult a qualified practitioner before taking anything in the first 3 months of pregnancy. Eat more wholemeal products, red kidney beans, liver, avocado, banana or Marmite or take Brewer's yeast. Alternatively, consult a qualified nutritional practitioner.

Meanwhile . . . where sickness is severe, lie down and keep perfectly still with a hot water bottle over your abdomen. Hang on in there — it'll soon be over. Most cases of morning sickness wear off between 12 and 16 weeks.

Heartburn
Generally this is more of a problem during the later weeks of pregnancy. Lying semi-propped up in bed and having a milk drink at bed time can help. Herbal remedies include meadowsweet made up as a tea and sipped on and off during the day. Aniseed, with mint or lavender added, may also be helpful. For further advice consult a herbal

practitioner. Avoid eating over-spiced foods and eat little and often.

Constipation
This is sometimes a problem during pregnancy due to the relaxing effects of circulating hormones on smooth muscle. The answer is to make sure you have a good wholemeal diet, with plenty of raw foods. Drink plenty of fluids. Lemon juice in hot water on rising is a good trick to try. Herbal remedies may help, but as it's wise to avoid any drugs, including laxatives, during pregnancy you should consult a herbal practitioner to make sure it is safe. A tip recommended in an article by antenatal teacher Liz Winkler in *Parents* magazine is to take half a dessertspoonful of linseed in a glass of lukewarm water. She also recommends yoga (see page 121). Drink two glasses of water and rest in the frog position for ten minutes.

Insomnia
This can be because of anxiety over the pregnancy, or simply because your increased bulk makes it difficult to get comfortable. Homoeopathic remedies include arnica, nux vom, carbo vegetabilis, aurum and ignatia. For further details consult a homoeopath. Aromatherapy may be helpful. Sprinkle one or two drops of oil of lavender, camomile, marjoram or clary sage in your bath. A foot or leg massage is soothing. Always work towards the heart. Avoid massage of the spine or abdomen after the first 3 months of pregnancy. Better still get your partner to give you a massage with warm oils — and sprinkle a few drops of one of the oils on your pillow at night.

Piles

You are less likely to get these if you are following the wholefood diet recommended. Sponging them with ice-cold water will bring relief, or sitting in a cold hip-bath. Itching can be relieved by bathing the haemorrhoids (to give them their proper name) in an infusion of chervil. It's best not to take herbs internally unless recommended by a qualified practitioner.

Yoga poses such as the Fish, Plough and Shoulder Stand can all benefit piles. Homoeopathic remedies include calcerea fluorata (for bleeding and itching), hamamelis (when oozing dark blood), ignatia — for painful protruding piles, and for itching again — nux vom.

Varicose veins

Some women develop varicose veins for the first time in pregnancy. Taking plenty of exercise, wearing special support tights, and sitting with your feet raised can all help. Much of the advice applying to piles, especially exercising, is useful here. A handful of dried marigold flowers steeped in a cup of witch hazel then applied to each leg with flannels can bring relief, or handbaths containing a mixture of hawthorn, broom flowers, yarrow and rose petals. For internal remedies consult a qualified herbalist.

Homoeopathic remedies include hamamelis in tincture form, carbo vegetablis to improve circulation, and after you've had the baby-pulsatilla.

High blood-pressure

Very high blood-pressure (over 140/90), especially if combined with protein in your urine, swelling, eyesight problems or headaches, needs medical attention either from an orthodox doctor or a medically qualified alternative practitioner. However, less severe blood-pressure problems can be successfully treated using relaxation techniques. In one study meditation combined with biofeedback was found to be successful in avoiding the need for hospital admission and bedrest in a group of women with mild high blood-pressure. High blood-pressure can be treated by cutting out tea and coffee and substituting a herb tea such as lime blossom instead. Footbaths of hawthorn, celandine and broom flowers with a head of garlic are recommended in *The Alternative Directory of Symptoms and Cures*, Dr Caroline M. Shreeve, (Century). Homoeopathy can also be useful, as can reflexology.

The Brewer diet is a high calorie diet devised by American nutritionist Tom Brewer which is said to prevent pre-eclamptic toxaemia (a disease of pregnancy involving the three symptoms of high blood-pressure, swelling and protein in the urine):

Each day:
— 4 glasses milk (2 pints)
— 2 eggs
— 3 servings fish, shellfish, turkey/chicken (4 oz per serving)
— 2 helpings of fresh green leafy vegetables.
— 5 servings bread, pasta, wholemeal cereal, brown rice
— 2 choices from whole potato, lemon, grapefruit, tomato, large glass fresh fruit juice
— 3 pats butter
— Salt to taste
— Fluids to taste
— 5 yellow or orange fruits or vegetables per week
— Liver once a week.

Follow the stress relieving measures described in part one, and pay attention to getting a good night's sleep.

Stretch marks

There's no sure way to avoid stretch marks, though not gaining too much weight and making sure you are not overweight to start off with may help. Some women have said the following aromatherapy remedy helps: 2 dessertspoonsful of wheatgerm oil added to a teaspoon of lavender oil in a cup of almond oil, massaged in every day.

Acupuncture for pregnancy and childbirth

Acupuncture can tune up your body so it is in the best possible shape to cope with pregnancy and childbirth, so it makes a useful adjunct to the types of pre-pregnancy care mentioned earlier. It can also help with morning sickness, urinary problems, high blood-pressure, swelling and fatigue. In the book *Birth Matters*, edited by Ros Claxton, natural healer Carol Rudd claims that acupuncture can be used to turn a baby in the wrong position, and during birth if the placenta fails to come away or if you develop post-partum haemorrhage (bleeding). This could be due to the effect acupuncture has on uterine contractions. A study carried out by a medical student under the auspices of the Centre for the Study of Alternative Therapies, looked at the possibility of inducing labour using electroacupuncture. In fact only one woman went into labour with acupuncture alone. However acupuncture did seem to increase the number and strength of contractions. Further studies are obviously needed to see how useful it might in fact be.

Yoga and pregnancy

Yoga is a particularly appropriate form of antenatal preparation, yoking as it does body, mind and spirit. Many women are now seeking out yoga preparation to childbirth, as an alternative to more traditional types of relaxation and breathing classes. And yoga plays an important part in many of the 'alternative' birth classes laid on by the Active Birth Movement.

It's a big subject, and if you are interested in finding out more, I'd advise you to read *Yoga and Pregnancy*, by Sophy Hoare, (Unwin). Here I'll just outline a few of the benefits to be gained from regular yoga practice during pregnancy. Opposite you'll see illustrated a few of the postures that might be especially useful.

Benefits of yoga during pregnancy

● **Physical benefits.** It helps you develop a strong supple body and back, so that you can bear the stresses and strains of pregnancy more easily. It helps with posture and so may alleviate backache and other aches and pains. It strengthens the body without tightening the muscles — this is important for birth.

● **Breathing.** Breath control exercises improve the oxygen flow in your blood and to and from the placenta. Learning to control your breathing is especially useful during labour. You can breathe more deeply or lightly to reduce pain from contractions and help you deal with pain. Smooth, calm breathing helps you relax and relieves anxiety.

● **Mental benefits.** Concentration and meditation can help you to focus in on yourself, a useful skill during labour when the sensations from the uterus can be

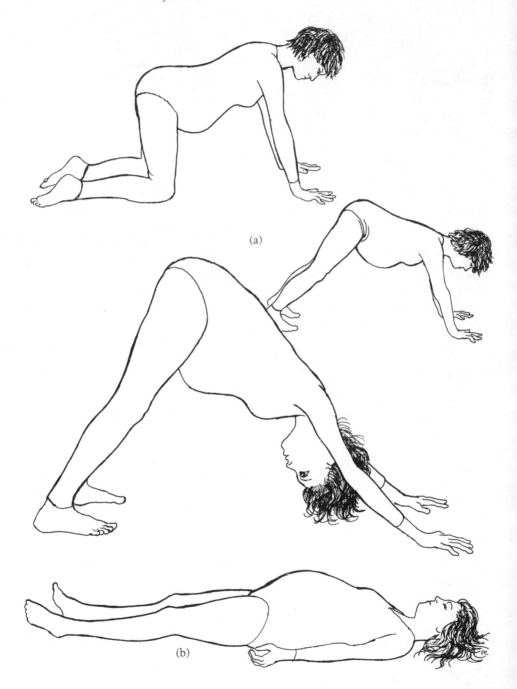

(a)

(b)

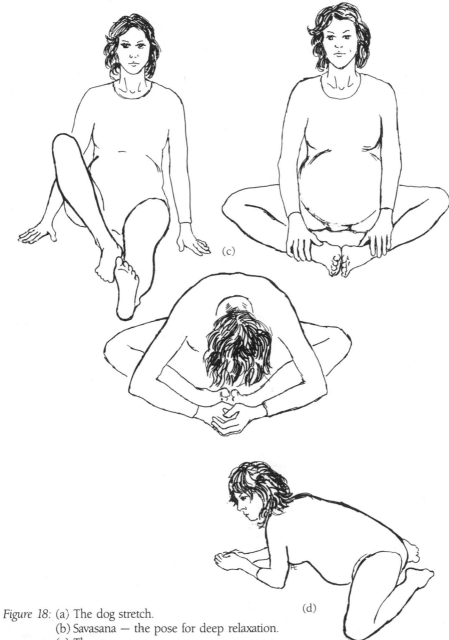

Figure 18: (a) The dog stretch.
  (b) Savasana — the pose for deep relaxation.
  (c) The star.
  (d) The frog.

overwhelming. This again can help with pain relief. More importantly, yoga can help you have confidence in the way your body operates, so that you are less likely to get frightened during labour. Experts have pointed to a strong connection between fear, tension and pain in labour. If you practise yoga regularly you'll be able to listen to your body and know instinctively what postures are most likely to help you during labour.

It's almost impossible to teach yourself yoga, so seek out a good yoga teacher.

After you have had your baby yoga can help relax you, and give you a calm centre in a life that has probably drastically changed. Sophy Hoare says in *Birth Matters:*

'To try to hold on to a fixed image of yourself leads to suffering when the image can no longer hold its own against reality; at the same time, behind ideas and images can be found the unchanging centre of the self when we are able to let go of our fixed attitudes and expectations. Yoga brings us in touch with the flow of life and with the enduring centre; in this way changes in our circumstances can be accepted without fear of losing our personal identity.'

Osteopathy for pregnancy

Osteopathy can be used in the pre-pregnancy period to help rebalance your body. It's especially useful for the problems caused by the changing weightload of your body which can cause backache and other aches and pains during pregnancy. Treating the back can increase blood flow to the pelvic area. Osteopathy can also be useful during labour itself, pressure at the base of the spine can help soothe pain, and techniques such as 'hanging' from a rope or pole — yes you did see right — can help stretch the lower part of your spine, which may relieve pain. After birth osteopathy can help re-align your pelvis and spine. The British School of Osteopathy now runs a special pregnancy clinic in London where for £70 (1986 price) you can have seven osteopathic treatments, in preparation for birth and delivery.

Birth — pain-relief

There's a vast amount written on birth, and there isn't really space here to do the subject full justice, so I plan to concentrate on alternative pain-relief for labour.

Most women would agree that labour is painful. Only an estimated five per cent of us get away with a completely painless birth. And the popular image of the primitive tribeswoman who squats casually and painlessly behind a bush to give birth is a fallacy. Orthodox medicine's answer to the problem of pain in labour is to do away with it, by giving drugs. Unfortunately all the pain-relieving drugs used during labour have quite serious disadvantages as you can see from the section on orthodox methods of pain-relief. At least one prominent obstetrician has expressed the opinion that the disadvantages of pethidine — still the most widely used painkiller in labour — outweigh its advantages. Epidurals can completely relieve pain. But, and it's a big but, a survey in 1982 that was carried out at London's Queen Charlotte's Maternity Hospital showed that having an epidural doesn't necessarily guarantee a happier experience of childbirth. In fact it may do the opposite. Of the 1000 women studied, those who had received an epidural were more dissatisfied with the experience of childbirth, both immediately afterwards and a year later, than women who had refused all analgesia and those who accepted simpler forms of pain-relief. What's more, epidural isn't freely available throughout the country, so even if you do decide you would like to try it, you may not be able to have one.

Supporters of the alternative birth movement that has grown up in the last few years point out that many women could do without pain-relief altogether, or reduce their need for it, if they are allowed to walk around and choose the positions that are most comfortable.

The whole issue of pain-relief in labour is a thorny one, because it is tied up with the question of who controls childbirth. Quite simply, giving a pain-relieving drug is something the medical staff can do to help you if you are in labour. You ring the bell for a nurse during labour and chances are she will offer you something for the pain. Your fear and need will have been interpreted as pain, and this in turn strengthens the conventional medical interpretation of that need as stemming from pain.

The fact is pain — isn't an objective fact. All sorts of other factors can affect it, such as being in unfamiliar surroundings, being stranded on your back and forced to stay in the same position, because you are wired up to a drip or monitor, and interventions such as acceleration (speeding up) of labour itself can all affect the amount of pain you feel. In Holland where the majority of births take place at home, only 5 per cent of women have pain-relieving drugs compared with 85 per cent in this country. Why? Assuming that Dutch women can't be endowed with more courage than we are, it could be that they accept pain as part of the process of giving birth whereas we are conditioned to believe that all pain should be removed. It could also have a lot to do with the circumstances of birth.

It's known that physical and emotional support during labour can reduce or even eliminate the need for other forms of pain-relief, partly because labour is likely to be shorter in these circumstances. Also the more relaxed you are the more efficiently your uterus operates. A telling piece of research compared the pain-relief given to 100 women delivering in a GP unit or at home, with that received by similar women in the local hospital. Thirty eight per cent of women having first babies and 84 per cent of those having second or subsequent deliveries in the GPU did without pain relieving drugs.

If you feel you would prefer the minimum of drugs and intervention, and so long as your pregnancy is straightforward, it might be worth considering a home delivery or delivery in a GP unit. If you do have to go into hospital make sure your wishes are written on your notes. This is where your assertive techniques come in too. Many alternative birth teachers offer assertiveness training as part of preparation for birth.

Alternative and self-help approaches to pain-relief in labour

● **Stay up and about.** The illustrations

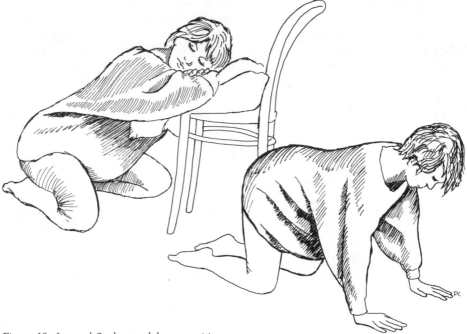

Figure 19: 1st and 2nd stage labour positions.

above show suitable positions for second and first stage labour. The more upright you can be, the stronger contractions are and the more effective, since the baby's descent is aided by gravity. An upright position also improves blood supply to the baby, so she is likely to be withstand the stress and strain of labour better, and less likely to get short of oxygen (become distressed).

● **Take a companion with you.** This could be your partner, a relative or friend.

● **Massage** will help ease pain. Low back massage using a firm circular motion, or get your partner to roll a tennis ball over your lumbar region, is very soothing. Effleurage — light fingertip massage — over your abdomen will be helpful too.

● **Make yourself at home** if you are going

into hospital. Take in something familiar that you like to look at such as a picture or vase of flowers. Having something to concentrate on such as a picture, a candle or a visual image can also help you focus inwards which in turn helps relieve pain.

● **Acupuncture** has been very successfully used to relieve labour pains, and caesarean sections have even been performed using acupuncture as the only anaesthetic. If you want to take an acupuncturist into hospital, it will be necessary to get the permission of your doctor. A pilot study carried out by a midwife in Glasgow and reported in *Midwives Chronicle,* May 1985 found that 75 per cent of women in labour who had received acupuncture said they would opt for it again next time they had a baby: 'common comments from the women in the study related to a feeling of "calmness" and the maintenance of self control during labour'.

● **Hypnosis** helps some women deal with labour pain, perhaps by easing tension. If you want to use hypnotherapy you should start to learn the necessary techniques from early on in pregnancy.

● **Herbal remedies** can be extremely effective in toning up your uterus in preparation for labour so that it is in the best possible shape. Raspberry leaf tea is one of the best known tried-and-tested remedies — you can drink it during the last three months (3 heaped teaspoons to a pot of tea taken two to three times a day). However it is probably best to consult a qualified herbalist before taking it, since raspberry leaves can tone up or relax the uterus. In some very athletic women the muscles of the uterus can become overtoned. Squaw vine (*mitchella repens*) is another useful remedy. Ros Claston and Carol Rudd recommend using aromatherapy oils such as rosemary oil or lavender and camomile during labour, either rubbed on to your forehead, wrists and neck or used in massage. You can also put a few drops of essential oil in a bowl of warm water and allow it to evaporate.

● **Homoeopathic remedies** include caulophyllum (which comes from the same plant as squaw vine) to tone up the uterus beforehand, and arnica which prevents and eases bruising. A homoeopath will be able to recommend other suitable remedies tailored to you as an individual for use during labour itself.

● **TENS** stands for transcutaneous nerve stimulation. It's an offshoot of acupuncture, and some acupuncturists believe it offers better pain relief than traditional acupuncture techniques, especially as some women dislike having the needles inserted during labour. Another advantage is that an increasing number of hospitals now have TENS equipment. TENS works by sending electrical impulses to the brain which block pain messages and stimulate the release of endorphins (the body's own pain relieving hormones). Incidentally this may be the key to how many alternative pain-relief methods work. The equipment consists of a small hand-held box with four electrodes which can be placed on particular acupuncture points on your back or abdomen. The sensation is one of vibration or pins and needles, which changes to a continuous electrical sensation. It's thought that TENS is successful in wiping out about 95 per cent of back pain during labour. And one midwife I spoke to reported that it could help some women to manage entirely without pain-relieving drugs. Others might need some pain-relief as a back up. But as one of a battery of other methods TENS certainly seems worth a try.

Orthodox methods of pain-relief

● **Pethidine.** Still the most widely used drug for pain relief, though it has been somewhat ousted in recent years by the epidural. It's given by injection. At its best it may make you feel relaxed and slightly woozy. But many women complain that it makes them feel drunk and out of control. It can also make you sick. The main disadvantage is that it crosses the placenta and babies exposed to large quantities tend to be drowsier and slower to suck. Some babies suffer breathing difficulties so another drug which reverses the effects of pethidine has to be given. In one study mothers who had had large doses of pethidine spent less time looking after and holding their babies in the hour after birth than a control group. This could be to do with the 'distancing' effect of the drug. Though it could also be argued that someone who had needed large amounts of pethidine might have had a pretty lousy labour anyway, and just want to rest after it all.

● **Epidural**. The only pain-relieving drug that can completely remove pain. It causes completely lack of sensation from the abdomen downwards, which some women find unpleasant. Drawbacks include the fact that once the epidural is in place (the drug is inserted via a catheter into the epidural space in your spine) you can no longer move around. What's more, if you have an epidural you'll be far more likely to have a very medically managed labour. You'll need to be electronically monitored since you won't be able to feel contractions. You may also need forceps delivery because unless the epidural is timed to wear off, you won't be able to feel the pushing sensations of second stage. Because of the paralysis of your pelvic floor muscles the new baby's head often doesn't rotate as it should — hence the need for forceps.

● **Gas and air.** Perhaps the most acceptable of orthodox pain-relieving methods. It's a mixture of nitrous oxide (laughing gas) and oxygen, you breathe it in at the start of each contraction. Pain relief is good, and because the gas passes out of your body between contractions there is less danger of it passing into your baby's system in large amounts. It seems to have less effect on the baby than pethidine and the level in your baby's blood falls rapidly as she begins to breathe.

After the birth — Getting back to normal

Stitches
If you've had stitches the following alternative remedies are useful:

● Arnica for bruising.

● Aim a warm hair dryer at the sore area.

● Cold ice packs against the stitches.

● Do your pelvic-floor exercises to stimulate circulation to the area to aid healing.

● Apply witch hazel and mix it with three parts water to soothe soreness.

● Calendula ointment can help too.

Breastfeeding
Success in breastfeeding depends on being able to feed your baby whenever she feels hungry, coupled with a good diet, sufficient rest and a large dose of confidence. Probably more women give up breastfeeding through lack of advice and support than for any other reason. However there are one or two specific problems that can be overcome using a mixture of self-help and alternative techniques.

Insufficient milk supply
Probably the most common reason women give for giving up breastfeeding. Make sure

you are eating a good wholefood diet, with plenty of fluids. Go for mineral water and fruit juices. Probably apple and grape are best as orange juice seems to disagree with some babies and make them colicky. Feed frequently. Milk supply relies on frequent stimulation of the nipples which stimulates hormones to send messages to the breasts to produce more milk. Goat's Rue (*Galega officinale*) (one or two tablespoonsful to a cup) made into a tea is a useful herbal remedy. Take it three times a day. For other remedies consult a qualified herbalist. Tension can interfere with your milk supply by inhibiting the 'let down reflex' which makes the milk flow out of your nipples, and sends messages to the breasts to produce more milk. Relaxation, yoga, meditation can all be good ways of relieving tension. There are numerous homoeopathic remedies to increase milk supply — these include *agnus castus*, asafoetida, causticum, pulsatilla, urtica urens. Consult a homoeopath for further advice.

Sore nipples

As well as being unpleasant in themselves, sore nipples can inhibit the milk supply by making you tense. Make sure your baby is properly on the breast. The whole of the nipple and the brown area (areola) around it should be in her mouth, and the nipple should be well back in the baby's mouth so it is not pressing on the hard palate. If your nipples do get sore, start feeding on the least sore side first. Expose your nipples to the air as much as you can. The air jet from a warm hair dryer or convector heater will aid healing. Allow a drop of breast milk to dry on the nipples, it contains a substance that helps healing. Honey, almond oil, calendula ointment can all be used. A chamomile based ointment called Kamillosan is readily available and very successful in treating sore nipples. Homoeopathic remedies include the good old faithful arnica, calendula as an ointment and/or taken internally, castor equi. graphites and chamomilla to mention a few. Consult a homoeopath for other ideas.

Postnatal depression

One study suggests that nearly 40 per cent of women suffer postnatal depression. More conservative estimates put the figure at 10-15 per cent. Even if you don't develop full blown depression, many women complain of chronic tiredness, and other niggling aches and pains such as backache, headaches, piles, period pains and coughs and colds — all of which have been associated with depression and certainly do nothing for mental well-being.

It's all a far cry from the rosy picture of motherhood that we get from the ad-men. The snag is even the experts haven't sorted out among themselves just what causes postnatal depression. Is it a true depressive illness? Is it sparked off by the hormonal upheavals of pregnancy and birth? Or does it arise out of the conditions of motherhood — the lack of recognition, isolation, and so on, that goes hand in hand with being a mother in our society. On the one hand we're told it's the most important job in the world, but all the 'rewards' which are traditionally allotted to valued jobs such as high pay, status and all the rest are noticeably missing. Vivienne Welburn, author of *Postnatal Depression*, (Fontana), who has herself suffered from it, told me:

'Postnatal depression is a result of all sorts of factors. Women are highly vulnerable and sensitive after having a baby and things affect them more than they would normally.'

In psychological terms, childbirth has been described as a 'crisis' — a major life event, which requires an enormous amount of readjustment. An Australian midwife and anthropologist speaking at the 1986 Marce Society conference pointed out that in closer-knit rural communities in undeveloped parts of the world, postnatal depression is unknown.

Orthodox treatment consists of anti-depressant drugs, hormones (Dr Katharine Dalton whose work on premenstrual tension I described earlier is the major proponent of this theory), and occasionally psychotherapy. The latest research is aimed at discovering which women are vulnerable to postnatal depression, with a view to intervening, by offering extra support and counselling.

What are the signs of postnatal depression?

Postnatal depression is different from fourth day 'blues', which most of us experience just after birth, and which does appear to have a strong hormonal connection. In fact depression may not be the main symptom at all. An unnatural high or excessive anxiety are both common. Postnatal depression sufferers will suffer some or more of the following: sadness, lack of self-esteem, loss of interest in former pleasures (such as food, sex, clothes), weepiness, despair, guilt, self reproach, exhaustion, lack of energy, irritability, inability to cope, feelings of isolation and withdrawal. You may experience fears connected with your baby's welfare, or alternatively be frightened that you are going to harm her.

Alternative treatments

Diet
Some interesting new research from the Department of Child Health at the Hospital for Sick Children in Bristol has looked at levels of vitamins B_2 (riboflavin) and B_6 (pyridoxine) in a group of 20 mothers suffering from postnatal illness. Half the depressed group were found to be lacking in B_2, while the depressed group had lower B_6 levels than a control group. Antibiotics and smoking had a marked effect on the levels of these vitamins.

Given that vitamin B_6 is especially susceptible to the effects of processing, it could be that many mothers who are depressed are simply not getting enough vitamins in their diet. The researchers also comment that 'more attention could be paid in this country to re-balancing vitamin levels and restoring gut flora after antibiotic treatment.' But they also suggest that the low vitamin levels could be a reflection of poor appetite in the depressed group. It looks as though it would be worth seeing a practitioner interested in nutrition before reaching for the anti-depressant bottle.

Herbalism and Homoeopathy
Many of the therapies suggested in the section on mental health are equally applicable to postnatal depression. Herbal treatments seem to work very well, with the emphasis being put on herbs that rebalance and integrate hormonal levels. Herbs such as skullcap and valerian may be used to alleviate depression and anxiety.

There are also a number of homoeopathic remedies which could be useful. In his book *A Woman's Guide to Homoeopathic Medicine*, Dr Trevor Smith (Thorsons), suggests a number of useful remedies, of which he says

Sepia is the most useful and should be used as a first line. The profile is 'weakness, sadness, and tiredness. A sense of indifference to everything and everybody is marked, together with obstinate constipation, constant hunger and a yellowish-brown facial discoloration.' For further details of the one that is right for you consult a homoeopath.

Finally, **Oestoepathy** seems to be useful in some cases of postnatal depression.

The Menopause

Menopause simply means the end of your periods. It can start as early as the 30's or as late as your 60's. It can also happen if for any reason you have to have your ovaries removed (oophorectomy). For most women it occurs between the ages of 45 and 55.

Like so many of the other conditions described in this book menopause is surrounded by myths. Like premenstrual syndrome and childbirth the problems many of us experience during the menopause are seen and treated as medical ones, when perhaps they can be better understood in relation to all the other things going on in our lives at the time. Menopause, for instance, often coincides with children leaving home, the loss of a spouse through divorce or death, the onset of ill health. All of which can cause stress. And as we've seen time and again now, stress can affect you and make any pre-existing symptoms worse. What's more, living in a culture where young is beautiful and older women are considered over the hill sexually can be enough to provoke depression and lack of self-esteem.

What signs and symptoms are associated with the menopause?

The catalogue of complaints makes depressing reading: vaginal dryness, hot flushes, night sweats, painful sex, dry skin, cramps, varicose veins, sore breasts, aches and pains in the joints, anxiety, depression, and brittle bones are the main ones. But even so, only some 10 per cent of women suffer really disabling symptoms according to the statistics, and chances are you might only experience one or two of these. Fortunately there are a lot of things you can do to help yourself.

Orthodox treatment

The familiar gamut of hormone treatment, tranquillizers and anti-depressants are orthodox medicine's answer to the problems of the menopause.

Hormone Replacement Therapy (HRT) is often prescribed, especially if you are troubled by hot flushes, the idea being that it is lack of oestrogen that causes flushing and vaginal changes. HRT is taken in pill form, rather like the contraceptive pill. A new development is an oestradiol skin 'patch' similar to the one discussed in the section on PMS. It consists of oestrogen with nowadays progestogen added, which means that you will get an 'artificial period' every month. The snag is we don't really know whether it is actually lack of oestrogen that causes the flushes. What's more there is disturbing evidence that HRT leads to increased incidence of cancer of the uterus and gall bladder problems. And we still have no idea of its long-term effects. You shouldn't have HRT if you suffer from liver problems, gall bladder disease, certain blood and circulatory disorders, fibroids or diabetes. And no doctor should prescribe it if you have a family history of breast cancer or cancer of the uterus. Even if you do decide to opt for HRT, don't expect it to work miracles, and aim for take the smallest possible dose for the shortest time possible.

Alternative therapies and self-help

Flushes and dry vagina
As you'd expect a good wholefood diet is the basis of an alternative approach. Some naturopaths recommend various supplements.

Supplements
Vitamin E can help an itchy dry vagina and hot flushes. Doses of between 200 IU and 600 IU a day are recommended. Experiment to find the lowest level that suits you. If it doesn't work straightway, don't give up — it can take three to four weeks to have an effect. Adding vitamin C and B and ginseng seem to improve its action.

A special word here should be made of *ginseng*, a herb which contains a number of substances that control the hormone levels in your body. In one Finnish study doctors found it helped dry vagina, hot flushes, sweats, tension, anxiety and palpitations. Take 600mg to 1200mg a day. It would probably be a good idea to consult a herbal practitioner in the first instance, since the quality of ginseng sold in health food shops varies a lot. While on the subject of *herbal remedies*, familiar raspberry leaf tea, cramp

bark, black cohosh and golden seal are all used. Passiflora tablets are useful if you are tense or anxious.

Vitamin F found in cold pressed oils such as olive oil, sunflower oil and linseed oil is said to help with skin problems and nervousness. Evening primrose oil may also help. Rina Nissim in *Natural Healing in Gynaecology*, (Pandora), recommends supplements of calcium, magnesium, iron and phosphorus. See the chart on pages 23-6 for naturally occurring forms of these. See a nutritional therapist for further advice. Exercise will help build up your bones and keep you supple. Swimming is a good one. The pelvic-floor exercises described in part one can help prevent prolapse and stress incontinence.

Regular sex, either with a partner or by masturbation, is one of the best treatments and preventive of menopausal problems, especially for lack of elasticity and dryness of the vagina. It also helps reduce stress. So go ahead and enjoy yourself! Aloe vera gel will lubricate your vagina if you have a tendency to dryness.

How to cope with hot flushes

● Follow the stress relieving measures suggested elsewhere in the book.

● Cool down with an ice-pack, iced water or freshen-up tissues.

● Avoid hot curries and too much spicy food.

● Cut out tea, coffee, alcohol, smoking and too much sugar.

● Wear cotton underwear and clothing and use cotton bed sheets to absorb sweat and make you feel more comfortable.

● Go for layers of clothing so you can strip down if you feel a flush coming on.

Osteoporosis (brittle bones)

Men and women experience bone loss from their late 30's onwards, but women, especially white small-boned women who live in Northern parts of the world are especially susceptible. Such women have less bone mass to start off with. You may also be especially at risk if you have at any time suffered from anorexia. What's more, women tend to get less exercise than men which can significantly reduce bone loss according to one study — which is one good reason to start exercising. After menopause, the amount of oestrogen secretion which affects bone loss is reduced. Something like 5 out of ten women will suffer osteoporosis after the age of 65 and a few will suffer very severely. Osteoporosis is responsible for the traditional dowagers, hump and the hip fractures that some older women seem prey to. Such problems can be prevented to some extent by getting plenty of calcium with vitamin D to aid absorption. There's evidence too that moderate weight-bearing exercise can be helpful. Experts say we need 700 to 1000mg of calcium a day before menopause, and 1000 to 1,500 thereafter. Vitamin D supplements aren't recommended for white women because of the risk of overdosing, except under the supervision of a qualified practitioner.

Making the best of calcium in your diet.
Eat a high fibre diet, but avoid adding extra bran since it contains phytic acid which can prevent calcium absorption. Alcohol, too, can interfere with calcium metabolism. Too much caffeine and salt can cause it to be excreted. Natural supplements such as dolomite and bone-meal are good sources of calcium. But, be warned — excess calcium can alter zinc, iron and manganese levels in the body which can spark off kidney stones. It's best, as with all supplementation, to seek the advice of a practitioner.

Hysterectomy

Although hysterectomies are performed on younger women, you're most likely to be given one if you are older. Hang on to your womb if you possibly can.

Good reasons to have a hysterectomy are:

● cancer of the cervix or lining of the womb

● large fibroids

● endometriosis or heavy persistent bleeding for any other cause

● disease of the ovaries and Fallopian tubes

● cancer of the uterus

● very occasionally, complications of childbirth

If you're offered a hysterectomy, discuss it very carefully with your doctor to ensure that it really is necessary. After the operation you may experience vaginal dryness, and will need time to recover. Not surprisingly, many women get depressed at the loss of their wombs. Acupuncture, reflexology,

(a)

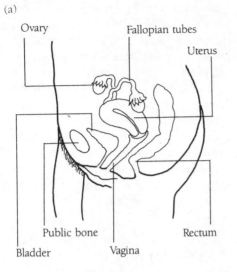

Ovary

Fallopian tubes

Uterus

Public bone

Rectum

Bladder

Vagina

(b)

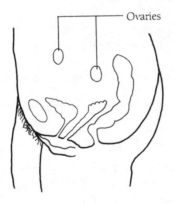

Ovaries

(c)

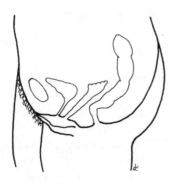

massage and homoeopathic and herbal remedies may all be helpful in the recovery period. You may also benefit from counselling or psychotherapy to help you come to terms with the operation. Any of the hands-on therapies or healing may be especially useful. A writer in *Nursing Mirror,* May 1985, describes how healing was stimulated by a nurse who held her head and put ice-packs on it: 'It may sound far-fetched, but I felt something in me respond to her touch, something which in the midst of all the pain, sweat and tears was the awakening of the will to recover.'

Further information:
Women on Hysterectomy
Nikki Henriques and Anne Dickson (Thorsons).
Older womens groups:
Womens Health Information Centre, 52 Featherstone Street, London EC1 (Tel: 01-251 6580).

Figure 20: Hysterectomy.
(a) Position of organs before hysterectomy.
(b) Removal of the uterus leaving the ovaries intact.
(c) Removal of the uterus and ovaries.

PART FOUR

The Therapies

Introduction

All the alternative therapies aim to treat you as a whole person, that is they are 'holistic', so any method of classifying them is going to seem a bit artificial. However, it's probably true to say that any one will take either the mind, body or spirit at a starting-point, though some such as yoga are so much total therapies that's it's hard to know which it acts on first. As you've read through the book you'll have got some idea of what the various therapies can do. In this section I try to give a brief run down of those mentioned elsewhere. You'll gradually get a feel for the therapy or combination of therapies that would best suit you. The tips I give are just starting-points, and if you feel inclined to try a particular therapy that appeals to you, don't be put off by the fact that I haven't recommended it for your particular complaint.

Alternative good, orthodox bad?

Alternative medicine has an appeal for women because it very obviously avoids some of the pitfalls outlined in section one. In our everyday lives we are used to being compartmentalized and fragmented, and alternative medicine may seem especially useful because it does aim to see people as a whole. An alternative practitioner will want to know all about you, where you live, what sort of foods you eat, the quality of your relationships, all about your work and the degree of satisfaction you feel with your life. Good healers of all types have, of course, always taken such factors into account.

Just as important, as we've seen throughout the book, the alternative therapies work by kicking the body's own defence system into action, rather than by suppressing or removing symptoms. This makes the alternative therapies especially suitable for so many of the conditions that are often defined as 'illness' by the medical profession, but which in actual fact are an integral part of our lives as women such as pregnancy, menstruation and the menopause.

> 'Health is restored by working in harmony with nature rather than against it.' Dr Alex Forbes, former director of Cancer Help Centre, Bristol.

But that's not to say that orthodox is all bad, or that alternative is bound to be good. For a start it's virtually impossible to get alternative treatment on the NHS which rules it out for many of us. And alternative treatment doesn't come cheap — in a recent survey carried out by *Which?* magazine October 1986, charges varied from £8 to £25. The cheapest treatment I could find was at the Women's Natural Health Centre, in Kentish Town, where treatment costs £6 or even lower if you can't afford that, but the clinic is intended only for those on a very low income. Given that the therapies tend to work slowly and gradually, even at the cheapest rates you could be letting yourself in for a pretty hefty bill.

The good news is that many more orthodox doctors are offering some form of alternative treatment. But some alternative therapists disapprove of this on the grounds that they may have only done a weekend course in a particular therapy, which they say is as bad as an alternative practitioner trying to remove an appendix after just such a course. A small number of practices actually employ alternative practitioners, as part of the health care team. But these are few and far between.

If you are hard up it's worth seeking out a practitioner who has a sliding scale of fees. Some of the alternative therapy organizations, such as the Medical Herbalists for instance, have training schools where you can get cheaper treatment for a student under supervision of a qualified practitioner. For further details of schemes contact the appropriate professional body. Another problem with alternative health care is that the majority of alternative practitioners are thin on the ground outside London and the home counties.

What's more, just because a treatment is 'alternative' doesn't mean it is necessarily safe, though the majority of them are, in the right hands. But there have been horror stories

of people getting seriously ill by following certain rigorous diet schedules for instance, or by taking too many supplements. However, it's important to keep the dangers in perspective — the orthodox medics are just as guilty if not more so of iatrogenic (doctor-caused) diseases.

The point is, it's just as important to be critical of alternative therapies as you would orthodox ones, and to choose your practitioner carefully. Make sure you understand your treatment and why it is being done. After all, you'd expect to know why you were taking a new powerful antibiotic, why not the same for a herb? The issue of self-help comes in here too. It is sometimes practical to treat minor ailments yourself using alternative methods, and throughout the book I've tried to indicate the sort of things you can do to help yourself. But, reading some of the books on alternative medicine on the market, you could be forgiven for thinking that you could treat almost any illness yourself using alternative therapies. Most alternative practitioners have to undergo lengthy training, and it would be just as unwise to think you could treat a complex illness such as cancer or endometriosis yourself without the guidance of a qualified alternative practitioner as it would without seeing a conventional doctor.

The BMA report published in 1986 criticizes alternative therapies on the grounds that they have been insufficiently tested. Many alternative practitioners would argue that the trial procedures appropriate to orthodox medicine, which treats symptoms rather than people, are simply not suitable to a group of therapies that start with the whole person. A conference laid on by the Research Council for Complementary Medicine, which includes both alternative and orthodox practitioners among its members brought out the need for new methods which take into account the unique action of alternative therapies, and which, contrary to orthodox medical trials, don't rule out the 'placebo' effect, which is an integral part of the body healing itself. This is going to be very difficult to organize since, for example, there may be an extremely large number of homoeopathic remedies suitable for any one set of symptoms, precisely because the remedy is matched to the patient rather than the disease. The good news is that the RCCM, the Institute of Complementary Medicine (ICM) and some of the alternative therapy organizations are beginning to make money available and set up their own trials.

But that's not all — naturopath Carol Smith, in an article in the magazine *Spare Rib*, warns against rejecting conventional scientific methods out of hand. If it hadn't been for studies and trials, for instance, many women would have continued to have radical breast surgery for cancers for which lumpectomy would have been just as good.

Another charge against alternative therapies is that because so much is laid at the door of lifestyle they can sometimes be guilty of more than a spot of victim-blaming. A medical herbalist writing in the journal *The Best of Health* says: 'Sometimes we *need* to be ill, have a headache, a day off work.'

All this is definitely not intended to put you off; merely to point out the need for a realistic approach.

Finding a therapist

Because the therapies are so diverse and there are no central training regulations as there are for conventional doctors it can be difficult to find an alternative practitioner. What should you be looking for? And how can you tell if he or she is any good?

Unfortunately there are no easy answers to these questions because so much depends on the individual. The advice to find out what works for you can be a costly and time-consuming business. And the advice to go to only a recognized or medically trained therapist is not as simple as it seems on the face of it either. Just as there are good and bad surgeons, there are good and bad lay-therapists, and good and bad medically trained ones. And as I said earlier, some doctors will have had only the skimpiest training in alternative techniques. In fact a survey carried out by the Threshold

Foundation some years ago found that half of all alternative practitioners are not registered with a professional association at all. Nonetheless, there are moves afoot to try and standardize training in each of the alternative therapies, and there is some suggestion that one way to achieve this would be for some sort of registration system, so you could ensure the person treating you was fully qualified. To this end several of the existing alternative medicine bodies have formed the Council for Complementary and Alternative Medicines.

Unfortunately, just to complicate matters, there's another such umbrella body called the Institute for Complementary Medicine, with the same aims and objectives but with a slightly different squint on the subject of alternative therapies. An article in the *Journal of Alternative Medicine* suggests that the main difference between the two is that the CCAM is keen to gain orthodox credence and so tends to stick to strictly scientific explanations of alternative therapies, while the ICM is more inclined to take into account the less acceptable 'spiritual' aspects of alternative therapies.

Another organization run by orthodox doctors, the British Holistic Medical Association, seeks to broaden treatment by encouraging orthodox medical practitioners to look into the various alternative therapies as an adjunct to conventional treatment. The BHMA has a number of local groups throughout the country where you can learn more about the various different types of therapy and how you can begin to take responsibility for your own health.

Checklist

To ensure you get a good therapist follow the tips below:

● Ask your doctor to recommend someone. The *Which?* survey mentioned above found that 9 out of 10 patients hadn't asked their doctor because they thought he would disapprove. But other research shows that G.P.s are often very interested in alternative therapies and many of them have tried one or several themselves. In any case it is a good idea to let your G.P. know if you are having some form of alternative treatment.

● Ask friends to recommend someone they have found helpful.

● Select a practitioner who is registered with one of the alternative professional organizations — at the moment this is your only safeguard that the practitioner you are going to has reached a certain standard.

● If you have a particular complaint, such as endometriosis, contact one of the self help organizations to see which therapies might be helpful.

● Join or form a self-help group (if there is a branch of the British Holistic Medical Association in your area this would be a good one) to find out what approaches are useful to your problem.

● Contact the practitioner you have chosen to see if s/he has treated your condition before. See if you can speak to people who have been treated to find out how satisfied they were.

● Don't expect miracles. Sometimes the best any practitioner can do is to help you live with your condition.

● Don't expect an instant cure. Most alternative therapies are gentle and take a while to work. The longer you've had a complaint the longer it will take to sort it out.

● Go for a practitioner who operates a sliding scale of fees. And find out beforehand how much you can expect to pay.

● Avoid practitioners who claim to have only one answer. A combination of approaches often works best.

● Avoid any practitioner who blames you for your illness.

● Look for someone you like and get on with, and who will listen to you and involve you with your treatment.

● Do remember orthodox medicine may be what is appropriate in your particular case. Alternative therapies seem to work best for chronic ailments, self-limiting illnesses and illnesses with a strong psychological component.

How can alternative therapies help?

1. They can help you stay well by drawing attention to effects of your life on your health (e.g. diet, exercise, stress).
2. They can help you deal with chronic disease and help alleviate some of the more troublesome problems.
3. If you get ill they can treat and even cure specific illnesses by helping to put the body's own self healing mechanisms into action.
4. By putting the emphasis on health rather than disease they can help you increase your sense of positive control over your life.

Further information:
The College of Health Guide to Alternative Medicine, Ruth West, £3 from the College of Health, 18 Victoria Park Square, Bethnal Green, London E2 9PF, Tel: 01-980 6263. The College also does a series of tapes on alternative therapies which you can listen to for just the cost of a phone call.

Healthline 01-980 9848.

The Centre for the Study of Alternative Therapies, 51 Bedford Place, Southampton SO1 2DG.

Women's Natural Health Centre
169 Malden Road
London NW5 4HA
01-267 5301

Research Council for Complementary Medicine
Suite 1
19A Cavendish Square
London W1M 9AD

British Holistic Medical Association
179 Gloucester Place
London NW1 6DX
01-262 5299

Institute for Complementary Medicine Yearbook, Directory of UK Practices, Therapies and Information, from the ICM, 2a Portland Place, London W1N 3AF. You can also contact their information service for advice and information about treatment but they won't usually give names of specific practitioners. Ring 01-636 9643.

A Woman's Guide to Alternative Medicine, Liz Grist, (Fontana).

The Alternative Health Guide, Brian Inglis and Ruth West, (Michael Joseph), comprehensive guide to therapies and treatment.

Alternative Medicine, Dr Andrew Stanway, (Penguin), A-Z of therapies.

Holistic Living: A guide to self care, Dr Patrick Pietroni, (Dent) Practical self help health guide by founder of British Holistic Medical Association.

The Alternative Dictionary of Symptoms and Cures, Dr Caroline M. Shreeve, (Century).

Nutritional therapies

In the last few years the orthodox medical world has begun to sit up and take notice of the role diet has to play in health. Following the publication of the NACNE and COMA reports on food and health, ideas that just a decade ago would have been dismissed as cranky or absurd have become part of the mainstream. It's surely a measure of how far we have come that an article on paleolithic diet (stone-age) based on wholefood principles should appear in the most prestigious medical journal *The New England Journal of Hospital Medicine.*

Naturopathy

Illness is seen by the naturopath as the body's effort to get back to normal. For this reason the naturopath won't attempt to suppress the symptoms of your illness. For example, if you have a temperature the naturopath will use techniques to encourage your body to sweat as a way to get rid of accumulated waste products.

The basic tenet of naturopathy is that a healthy diet and lifestyle can help prevent much illness occurring in the first place, and that if illness does occur such principles will allow the body's own restorative processes to get to work. According to the naturopath the basic causes of disease can be divided into three groups:

1. *Chemical.* Nutritional deficiency or excess can lead to imbalances in the body fluids leading to poor functioning of lungs, kidneys, bowels or poor circulation of body fluids.
2. *Mechanical.* Tight muscles, strained ligaments and stiff joints or poor posture perhaps because of work, or because the spine is out of balance, lead to problems of functioning for the nervous system and musculo-skeletal system.
3. *Psychological.* Stress leads to problems which can affect the whole body.

The naturopath stimulates the body to heal itself by helping it to get rid of poisons that may have built up. S/he also seeks to help you understand why you became ill in the first place so that you can take more responsibility for your own health and avoid, where possible, the things that have caused

you to become ill. Your first visit to a naturopath will probably be much along the lines of a visit to an orthodox doctor, except that it will be much longer. Blood tests, X-rays, as well as more unconventional methods of diagnosis such as kirlian photography, radionics, iridology and other more unusual techniques may be used.

Treatment may include one or more of the following:

● *A fast,* designed to clear out wastes. This should only ever be carried out under supervision.

● *A diet* consisting largely of raw foods, unrefined carbohydrates and a small amount of protein. This may be a type of vegetarian diet, depending on your therapist.

● *Hydrotherapy* — literally water-treatment. This can include applications of hot and cold water, either externally or internally in the form of baths, packs, compresses, sprays and douches, or sitz-baths (hip) in which the lower half of the body is immersed in hot or cold water, while the feet are put in water of a contrasting temperature.

● *Structural adjustments* by means of osteopathy, chiropractic, remedial exercises, or body realignment techniques such as Alexander Technique.

● *Natural hygiene* i.e. taking care of yourself by physical exercise, relaxation techniques and a positive approach to life.

Naturopathy can be used for virtually any condition, either as a mainstay or as an adjunct to other forms of treatment. It corresponds in many ways to the general principles for taking care of yourself outlined in the first part of this book.

Further information:
British College of Osteopathy and Naturopathy, 6 Netherhall Gardens, London, NW3 5RR. Tel: 01-435 8728. For £1 you can get a register of practitioners (enclose s.a.e.)

Naturopathic Medicine: Treating the Whole Person, Roger Newman Turner, (Thorsons).

Megavitamin Therapy/Optimum Nutrition

As we've seen throughout the book, many alternative practitioners believe that a large number of illnesses and disorders are a result of excesses or deficiences of certain important vitamins and minerals. It's important to get the right amount for you personally, since people's needs vary. Megavitamin therapy is said to be especially useful for all those vague aches and pains, chronic tiredness, lack of energy that afflict so many of us today, as well as menstrual problems, cancer and even mental disorders.

Patrick Holford of the Institute for Optimum Nutrition, 5 Jerdan Place, London SW6 1BE Tel: 01-385 7984 believes most of us could benefit from taking a daily multivitamin and mineral supplement. You can get such a pack from: Health Plus, 118 Station Road, Chinnor, Oxon OX9 4EZ — at the time of writing the cost is £7.95 plus postage.

Further information:
The Whole Health Manual, Patrick Holford, (Thorsons).
The Vitamin Bible, Earl Mindell, (Arlington).

Symbiosis therapy

Widely practised throughout Germany and Scandinavia. Health and illness are seen as two complementary aspects of life (rather like the yin and yang principle). It's when the 'dysbiotic' state caused by abnormal bacteria in the colon, overrides the natural balance of micro-organisms in the body that disease occurs. Disease such as irritable bowel syndrome, and candida (see page 66) are said to be the result of this. Treatment is through detoxification, rebalancing the acid-alkali level in the body, increasing circulation, and nutrition and breathing techniques. Probiotics aim to encourage the growth of 'good' micro-organisms, for example in the gut.

Further information:
The International Institute of Symbiotic Studies, 5 Fairlight Place, Brighton, BN2 3AH Tel: 0273 695880.

Clinical ecology

This is one of the fastest growing new approaches and in many ways forms a bridge between alternative and orthodox methods. The idea is that many of us are allergic to certain foods and chemicals. Because of the increased use of chemicals in food, and in the environment, such allergic illnesses are thought to be on the increase. These can be responsible for a wide range of conditions, including the everyday aches and pains such as excessive fatigue, irritability, and so on, that all too many of us take for granted, like migraine, bladder problems, thrush, and certain psychological disorders.

A major problem, according to clinical ecologists, is 'masked or hidden sensitivity', in other words most of us don't have any obvious reaction to the offending substances. It's only after a fast that a rapid and often dramatic reaction can be provoked. What's more, claim such practitioners, most of us are hooked on the very foods that are making us ill.

Diagnosis involves fasting, followed by a rotation diet in which foods are reintroduced one by one to spot the offending one. Other techniques include doing a white blood cell count, putting minute dilutions of particular foods in drops beneath the tongue, skin testing, muscle testing, and electrical testing.

Treatment consists of cutting the offending substances from your diet, putting you on a rotational diet in which such foods are only taken every few days, and desensitization.

There simply isn't space here to go into much detail about this fascinating new field.

Further information:
The Food Allergy Plan, Dr Keith Mumby, (Unwin).

The section on Clinical Ecology in *Alternative*

Therapies, edited by George Lewith, (Heinemann) is also very useful.

Action Against Allergy, 43 The Downs, London, SW20 will give advice and put you in touch with a doctor dealing in allergies.

Environmental Medicine Foundation, 10 St John's Road, Boxmoor, Hemel Hempstead, Herts HP1 1JR. Tel: 0442 58112.

National Society for Research into Allergy, PO Box 45, Hinkcley, Leicestershire, LE10 1JY.

British Society for Clinical Ecology, Dr Michael Radcliffe, Hythe Medical Centre, Hythe, Hampshire. He will let your doctor have a copy of a list of qualified doctors practising clinical ecology.

British Society for Allergy and Environmental Medicine, Acorns, Romsey Road, Cadnam, Southampton SO4 2NN Tel: 0703 812124.

Herbalism

Herbs have been used for medicine throughout the ages and in every culture. The Chinese, Indians and North Americans all have well developed forms of herbal medicine, and indeed the orthodox pharmocopeia includes many drugs which have their origins in herbs. Herbalism also seems to have a particular attraction for women, perhaps because, as Barbara Ehrenreich and Deirdre English point out in *Witches, Midwives and Nurses: a history of women healers* (Writers and Readers): 'Women have always been healers . . . They were pharmacists, cultivating healing herbs and exchanging the secrets of their uses. They were midwives travelling from home

to home and village to village. For centuries, women were doctors without degrees, barred from books and lectures, learning from each other, and passing on experience from neighbour to neighbour and mother to daughter.'

Because herbs are there for the picking in every field and hedgerow it is tempting to treat yourself. And it's true that herbal remedies can provide simple self-help treatments for many minor ailments, *if you know what you are doing*. If you are interested in pursuing this I'd advise you to get hold of Barbara Griggs, *The Home Herbal*, published by Pan. But for anything that doesn't clear up quickly that you would normally take to the doctor, you would be unwise to try and treat yourself

After all you wouldn't try to take your own appendix out would you? Herbal practitioners undertake a complex 4-year training. They need to know not just the symptoms and treatment of illnesses, but which particular herb to use, what part (leaves, berries, root, bark), how to prepare and apply it, even what time of day to harvest it. Judgement is also needed as to how much to give. Even conventional medicines affect two different people differently, and this is even more marked with herbs. It's far too important a decision to be left to guesswork. Remember too, that if you're already taking a precribed or over-the-counter remedy the herbal treatment could well affect its action in some way.

Herbal treatments work on you and not just on your symptoms, so two entirely different remedies might be given to treat the same disorder. That's why although I've included a few self-help tips throughout the book, you would be advised to consult a proper herbalist.

Herbal treatments are extremely effective because unlike orthodox drugs which take one active ingredient and synthesize it, the whole plant is used. So, while conventional diuretics for instance rob your body of potassium, creating other imbalances in your system, dandelion, a frequently used herbal diuretic contains large amounts of potassium to counterbalance this effect. Herbal treatments, unlike modern drugs which are aggressive in their action, are gentle. They provide trace elements, vitamins as well as active ingredients for a particular condition, which help you to return to full health. So whereas you may feel run-down and washed-out after a conventional course of treatment, after a herbal treatment you may feel full of energy.

What happens when you visit a herbalist?

The herbalist will take a long time to explore not just the illness you are going with, but your past medical history, too. If necessary, a physical examination will be carried out. And routine tests such as blood pressure, haemoglobin, urine test, will be done, just as if you were visiting an orthodox doctor.

By and large you will then be given a tincture, or syrup. But occasionally you will be given dried herbs to make up as an infusion (tea), decoction, or tablets or capsules. Poultices, ointments, lotions may also be prescribed for external use.

How long will it be before I get better?

Herbal remedies will often sort out a problem quickly. Where you have a long-standing problem it may take several weeks or months to clear. In the meantime you will be prescribed remedies to control the symptoms while the longer term treatment is taking effect. In extreme cases where surgery is unavoidable, for example if you have a severe prolapse, the herbalist may suggest this course of action.

What disorders can herbalism treat?

Most women's ailments can be successfully treated by herbal methods. Painful periods, heavy and irregular periods can all be helped. A course of the appropriate medicine will be used with extra medication during your period at first. Where a hormone imbalance is suspected of being the cause herbs will be used to correct it, and in this case treatment will probably go on for about six months. There are no side-effects and you will usually notice some improvement after one or two cycles. Premenstrual syndrome is very well treated by herbs, and usually needs about 6-12 months treatment consisting of one dose of medicine a day. Migraine associated with PMS takes a little longer to sort out, but results are good. Vaginal infections are successfully treated using a combination of medicine, pessaries or lotions plus making dietary changes.

Infertility can in some cases be treated, where for instance there is a hormone imbalance causing hostile mucus, endometriosis or pelvic infection. Problems of the menopause such as hot flushes, night sweats, dry vagina and so on can be treated, again by helping the body adjust to changes in hormones that may lie behind such problems. Mastitis, cystitis, irritable bladder can all be treated. For bladder problems, soothing and antiseptic herbs are used, often in the forms of herb teas, since tea and coffee act as irritants. Herbs can also treat many of the minor ailments of pregnancy safely. and raspberry leaf tea is famed for its effect on toning up the uterus in preparation for labour. Post-natal depression can also be helped.

Where can I find out more?
Write to the National Institute of Medical Herbalists, 41 Hatherley Road, Winchester, Hants, for a list of qualified practitioners. (Enclose large s.a.e) Members of the Institute carry the letters MNIMH or FNIMH after their name.

To make a herbal compress
Use a clean muslin or cotton cloth and soak in a hot infusion or decoction. Place it on the affected area and change it when it cools down.

A poultice is similar to a compress except that you use the plant itself. Place either fresh or dried herbs between some muslin and apply to the affected part. Dried herbs should first be made into a paste using hot water.

Using a herbal douche
Buy a douche from Boots, or if you can't get one, get a disposable one and discard the contents, wash it out well. Use an infusion or decoction that has been allowed to cool. Pour into the container and insert the applicator into your vagina. This will be easier if you are sitting on the lavatory, since the contents will run out. Use three times a day for seven days. If the condition has not improved in this time see a qualified practitioner.
NB. **NEVER douche if you are pregnant**.

Aromatherapy

The use of essential oils derived from aromatic plants and trees for healing. There are about 60 main oils in common use. The oils are either taken by mouth, or they may be added to your bathwater, used for massage, inhaled or given as compresses, douches or enemas. It's especially useful for stress-related illnesses, either as an adjunct to conventional or alternative therapies or used alone. Some practitioners discourage taking the oils by mouth because it is thought they may harm the mucus lining of the gullet and digestive tubes. It's best not to treat yourself, but to consult a qualified practitioner.

Further information:
The Power of Holistic Aromatherapy, Christine Stead, (Javelin). Useful self help guide for number of minor ailments.

The Use of Essential Oils and *Health and beauty,* Daniele Ryman (Winward).

London School of Aromatherapy, 42a Hillfield Park, London N10 3QS

Essential oils are available from:
Neal's Yard Apothecary,
2 Neal's Yard
Covent Garden
London WC2

Potters Ltd
Leyland Mill Lane
Wigan
Lancs WN1 2SB

Culpeper   .
Hadstock Road
Linton
Cambridge
CB1 6NJ

Bach Flower remedies

Dr Edward Bach believed that the cause of any physical illness was a negative emotional state. He claimed that by working on these emotional states by means of the essential energy in certain flowers many physical ailments could be overcome. Method of preparation involved 'placing the flower heads on the surface of water in a plain glass bowl in full sunlight for three hours,' then bottling it. The 38 remedies which you can get from a health food shop are dropped into water and drunk. It all sounds fantastic but one practitioner who uses Bach Flower remedies in conjunction with counselling, reflexology and visualization techniques claims they can be a useful back-up to these other methods. Because they are completely harmless they can be safely used for children and babies. A useful remedy is the Rescue remedy, a combination of five Bach Flower remedies used for 'panic, shock, sorrow, terror, sudden bad news and accidents'.

Homoeopathy

Homoeopathy is one of the most intriguing and yet mystifying of all the alternative therapies. It's the only 'alternative' available on the NHS, and there are five homoeopathic hospitals in London, Glasgow, Liverpool, Bristol and Tunbridge, operating mainly on an outpatient basis. If you want to visit one of these you'll need a letter from your G.P., or a medically qualified homoeopath.

Homoeopathy works on the principle of 'like cures like'. Remedies made from natural substances such as herbs, salts, minerals, and even diseased tissue or discharges (nosodes), are used in microscopic dilutions. The idea is that giving minute doses of a medicine that would in a healthy person produce the symptoms of the illness being treated, stimulates the body's own curative processes. And if that sounds crazy think of X-rays which are known to both cause and cure cancer or vaccines, which raise resistance to the illness in question.

There are various homoeopathic first-aid and self-help remedies, and any of the suppliers listed will be happy to provide lists of the most common ones. However, like herbalism, it would be unwise to try and treat yourself for any but the most simple ailments. There are several books on the market at the moment, which give listed remedies for various women's ailments. In my opinion these are too confusing and worse than useless to the uninitiated. Homoeopathic remedies are prescribed for the individual. A homoeopath will spend a great deal of time building up a detailed total picture of you as a person and your particular symptoms.

What happens when you visit a homoeopath?

Expect to spend about an hour and a half on your first consultation. The homoeopath will take a careful history of your symptoms, but will also ask you what you might consider to be some pretty strange questions, such as 'Do you prefer to be by the seaside or up in the mountains?' 'What sort of weather do you prefer?' She'll also want to know about your family medical history and will ask you about events in your emotional life, such as whether you have suffered a bereavement and how it affected you. She'll want details too about outside factors that affect your symptoms — for instance, is your illness better for warmth or cold? All these seemingly unrelated factors are taken into account when prescribing a remedy.

How long will it be before I get better?

Sometimes a single remedy will clear up not just the signs and symptoms of the illness you have gone to the homoeopath with, but of other ailments or conditions you might not have mentioned. A homoeopath told me the story of a woman who had gone complaining of tennis elbow, two weeks afterwards she rang up to say that a splinter of glass that had been in her skin for two years had worked its way out too. Sometimes there may be temporary worsening of your condition before you experience any improvement. This is considered to be a sign that the remedy is working. In the case of a long standing illness it may be necessary to continue giving the same treatment for some time, or to change the remedy to treat different symptoms. In cases where irreversible bodily changes have already taken place other types of treatment or even surgery may be advised, followed up by homoeopathy.

What disorders can homoeopaths treat?

Homoeopathy can successfully treat most women's ailments, even cysts and fibroids, though these may need surgery. Some cases of cystitis and vaginal discharge may need antibiotics or conventional treatment. But homoeopathy may be especially successful for bladder infections that have proved resistant to conventional treatments. Menstrual problems, headaches and problems associated with the menopause can also be treated, as can stress-associated states such as anxiety and depression.

Treatment is in the form of slightly sweet pleasant-tasting pills, powders or drops. There are homoeopathic ointments and creams for external use.

How does it work?

Sceptics always ask how can such infinitesimal doses work. The short answer is: we don't know. Clinical trials of homoeopathic treatment are exceptionally difficult to design, since the same illness will need different remedies depending on the person. However homoeopathy does seem to work, even for children and animals, where the 'placebo effect' is hardly likely to account for improvements.

The answer may lie in electromagnetic fields — but so far this hasn't been proved.

Homoeopathy and women

It has to be said that because homoeopathy depends so much on subjective views of individuals, there can be a danger of stereotyping, which can affect women. Homoeopaths sometimes speak of their patients in terms of their remedies. You'll hear them saying, 'She's a typical Pulsatilla',

for instance. And because many of the materia medica (the books containing symptoms and remedies used by homoeopaths for prescribing) were formulated sometimes a hundred years ago, the views of women can be sexist to say the least. Homoeopathic literature makes fascinating reading, but it's also full of descriptions that make your hair curl. Take these from a recent book on alternative therapies written for doctors:

'Lycopodium patients are usually intellectual, and capable, often lawyers, accountants or doctors. They worry excessively and anticipate events, having an anxious frown and often suffer from dyspepsia or an ulcer. The housewife who is tried, irritable, weepy and has lost interest in her home and family will often respond to Sepia.'

Sexism rules OK? It's especially important when choosing a homoeopathic practitioner therefore to find out whom you like, and who shares your views.

Further information:
Medical doctors with homoeopathic training will have MFHom after their names. You can get a list from The British Homoeopathic Association, 27a Devonshire Street, London W1 (s.a.e. essential). Lay homoeopaths will be registered with the Society of Homoeopaths, who run 4-year courses: 11a Bampton Street, Tiverton, Devon.

Using homoeopathic remedies

● For self-help for everyday ailments take the 6th potency.

● For acute conditions take every two hours for two days, then three times daily between meals for 3 days.

- For chronic conditions take 3 times a day between meals until you feel relief. When you feel some improvement decrease the number of doses, and stop altogether once you have felt significant improvement.

- Store medicines away from direct light, and strong smelling substances such as toothpaste, perfume, disinfectants.

- Take medicines in a 'clean' mouth. Allow half an hour after eating or cleaning your teeth or smoking a cigarette.

- Don't handle tablets and if any are spilled don't re-use them.

Biochemic Tissue Salts

German homoeopathic physician Dr W. H. Schuessler put forward the view that disease was linked to an imbalance of essential minerals. He believed that the body contains 12 essential minerals salts, if these become imbalanced disease results. A dose of the appropriate remedy restores health. The 12 Tissue Salts are available from most health food stores and can be used for self help. Instructions are usually given on the container and they are quite easy to use. The twelve salts are as follows:

1. Calcium Fluoride (Calc. Fluor.)
2. Calcium Phosphate (Calc. Phos.)
3. Calcium Sulphate (Calc. Sulph)
4. Phosphate of Iron (Ferr. Phos.)
5. Potassium Chloride (Kali Mur.)
6. Potassium Phosphate (Kali Phos.)
7. Potassium Sulphate (Kali Sulph.)
8. Magnesium Phosphate (Mag. Phos.)
9. Sodium Chloride (Nat. Mur.)
10. Sodium Phosphate (Nat. Phos.)
11. Sodium Sulphate (Nat. Sulph.)
12. Silicic Oxide (Silica)

The tissue salts are all given in a minute dose just as in homoeopathy and selection of the remedy is similar though simpler.

Further information:
Biochemic Handbook, Colin B. Lessell, (Thorsons).

Hands-on therapies

Osteopathy
Invented by Dr Andrew Taylor Still in 1874, osteopathy involves correcting structural defects in the spine to stimulate healing. The idea is that structural problems such as misalignment of the bones in the spine, muscle spasm and so on affect nerve and blood flow to other areas of the body, which if prolonged can result in disease. Treatment consists of setting right these defects by means of thrusts, stretching, massage and a variety of other neuromuscular techniques designed to relax the muscles and ligaments.

Osteopathy is widely accepted by

orthodox medicine as a treatment for back pain, and other discomfort. It can also be used for a whole variety of other illnesses, including migraine, constipation, period pains and digestive disorders. Osteopathy may be especially useful for a number of complaints affecting women by freeing blood flow to the pelvic area. The British School of Osteopathy has a special pregnancy clinic as already mentioned in the pregnancy section of the book, with an osteopath specially trained in gynaecology and obstetrics in attendance.

Visiting an osteopath

When you go to see an osteopath he'll be looking out for clues to the underlying cause of your complaint. He'll take especial note of your posture and the way you move. He'll want details about your life and work in order to see if these are causing any particular stresses and strains. The detailed medical history is followed by a physical examination of your spine. Osteopaths are extremely skilled at detecting the minutest imbalances in spinal structure. If necessary X-rays, urine or blood tests will also be used to aid diagnosis.

Apart from specific osteopathic treatment, the osteopath will give you advice on exercise and how to use your body to maintain health.

Cranial Osteopathy

A very gentle technique which involves exploring the pulse of cerebrospinal fluid by means of gentle pressure on the skull and in the pelvic area. It can be used to treat migraine, and babies who have had a difficult birth often benefit from it.

Further information:
British Naturoapthic and Osteopathic Association, 6 Netherhall Gardens, London NW3 5RR.

British Osteopathic Association, 8-10 Boston Place, London NW1 6HQ. Tel: 01-262 5250.

British School of Osteopathy, General Council and Register of Osteopaths, 1-4 Suffolk Street, London SW1Y 4HG.

Chiropractic

Like osteopathy, chiropractic involves manipulating and adjusting the spine and other joints. The basis of it is that the spine protects the spinal cord. If the spine is not in proper alignment it interferes with the nerve supply, so that the body cannot function properly. The result is disease.

Chiropractic is useful for a whole range of complaints. Like osteopathy the most common ones to be treated are back pain, neck problems and headaches. A recent study by one of the professional chiropractors' associations showed that patients had also been helped with menstrual problems, insomnia, constipation, bladder problems. The same survey reported that 80 per cent of patients got some help from the treatment.

What happens when you visit a chiropractor?

This is very similar to an osteopathic consultation. The chiropractor will take a full case history and may use X-rays to aid diagnosis. A physical examination to detect specific misalignments is next. Treatment consists of thrusting directly on certain bones, a process called adjustment, with a view to encouraging them to return to their correct positions.

What is the difference between chiropractic and osteopathy?

While the osteopath treats structural imbalances by means of levering and twisting the body, the chiropractor treats the bones separately by means of specific thrusts.

Further information:

The British Chiropractic Association, 5 First Avenue, Chelmsford, Essex CM1 1RX.
You can get 8 leaflets dealing with a number of common complaints such as back pain, by writing to the above enclosing a 9×6 inch s.a.e.

The Institute of Pure Chiropractic, (McTimoney Chiropractors) PO Box 126, Oxford, OX1 1UF.
This is an especially gentle type of chiropractic manipulation. The institute also has a number of training clinics offering reduced rates.

Touch for health — Applied Kinesiology

One of the fastest growing therapies in the UK at the moment. Anyone can learn a few basic principles that can then be used as a preventive. It's based on special techniques designed to test the muscles for areas of weakness. The technique forms a link between the traditional ideas of energy flow (chi) familiar from oriental therapies such as acupuncture and acupressure, and chiropractic.

A practitioner will take a case history and then examine you, usually lying down, for areas of muscular weakness. These can then be treated using pressure on the appropriate points. The idea is to restore balance rather than treating individual weaknesses. Applied kinesiology is also used as a diagnostic method in other alternative therapies, such as chiropractic and clinical ecology.

Further information:
British Touch for Health Association, Charles Benham, Information Officer, 29 Bushey Close, High Wycombe HP12 3HL.

Acupuncture

Not so long acupuncture was viewed with the utmost distrust. Today of all the alternative therapies it's the one that seems to be attracting the most serious medical interest. There are two types of acupuncture being carried out in this country: the traditional Chinese variety, and the modern 'scientific' type which relies on scientific explanations of its mode of action.

Chinese medicine, in which acupuncture has its origins, believes that health consists of the balance between two opposing forces:

Yin (which corresponds to passivity or water) and Yang (which corresponds to activity and is represented by fire). For most of us the balance is not perfect — one day we feel fighting fit, the next a bit under the weather. Such change is normal. But if the balance in our bodies is seriously disturbed we're in trouble and we get ill. Acupuncture consists of righting the balance between Yin and Yang by stimulating acupuncture 'points' with fine needles. These points lie along invisible lines, meridians or channels which

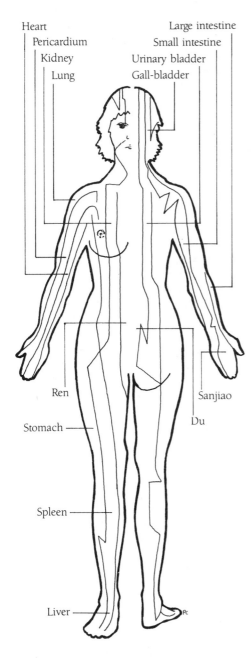

Heart
Pericardium
Kidney
Lung
Large intestine
Small intestine
Urinary bladder
Gall-bladder
Ren
Stomach
Spleen
Liver
Sanjiao
Du

Figure 21: The major accupuncture meridians.

are said to conduct vital energy or 'chi' through the body. All this might seem like so much mumbo-jumbo to Western ears, and the idea of chi is hard to explain. Basically it's a bit more than 'energy' but a bit less than matter. Blood, food and gases can be seen as material forms of chi.

Where women's health is concerned, then acupuncture can be especially important according to this view. In Chinese medicine for instance there's a condition known as 'empty blood' which can lead to period problems and depression. Treatment is by means of stimulating points that influence the blood, in order to increase production and aid flow.

Unexpressed emotions or emotional stress are recognized to affect physical problems. A classic acupuncture text *The Nei Ching* says that great grief, anxiety or overthinking will cause a tumour (cancer). Recent scientific thinking about immune mechanisms and their relation to stress is moving conventional medicine nearer to this approach.

However, the theories that have really led to acupuncture being taken into the fold are to do with its pain-relieving effects. It was found in the 1970's that stimulation of the acupuncture points resulted in the release of endorphins, the body's own pain relieving substances. Other theories have surmised that acupuncture works by stimulating large nerve-fibres which blocks the pain impulses carried by small nerve fibres (Gate Control Theory). Acupuncture also seems to have a striking effect on the autonomic nervous system. And some recent research points to its anti-inflammatory effect, which could account for its success in treating conditions such as arthritis.

Not all acupuncturists use the traditional

system of point selection. Instead, they treat tender points on the skin arising from musculo-skeletal problems. Surprisingly these points seem remarkably similar to the traditional acupuncture channels.

Diagnosis and treatment

The acupuncturist will spend time taking a detailed life history, taking note of such factors as your constitution, your emotions, and so on. You'll then be examined to see where any imbalances may lie. On the basis of this he or she will select the appropriate points. Treatment consists of placing needles in these points which remain there for anything from a few seconds to an hour. Sometimes a low level electric current is applied to the needles, which is thought to encourage endorphin release. It doesn't hurt, though you will probably experience a dull, numb feeling or a tingling sensation up and down the meridian.

Symptoms usually disappear gradually though some people get instant improvement. More likely though, your condition may get temporarily worse. No need to worry about this, it's a sign that your body is responding to treatment.

Acupuncture is now available in three quarters of the specialized pain clinics in this country, which is its main use within orthodox medicine. It's been found to be effective for 60 per cent of chronic pain sufferers which makes it specially useful for conditions such as endometriosis, headaches, period pains. It can also be used for childbirth and stress-related disorders such as depression.

There are three types of acupuncturists — medically qualified ones, lay therapists and physiotherapists who have taken a course in acupuncture. If your doctor isn't trained he can refer you to a lay therapist though he still retains overall responsibility for your treatment.

Ear acupuncture (Auricular acupuncture)

Parts of the ear are said to correspond to different organs in the body. So, for instance if you have a pain in your hand you will experience a pain when the part of your ear corresponding to the hand is pressed. In 70 per cent of cases reported in one study pain could be identified in this way. See diagram of ear acupuncture points on page 153.

Further information:
British Medical Acupuncture Society, 67-9 Chancery Lane, London WC2A 1AF (will send a list of members, but you'll have to be referred by your G.P.)

The Council for Acupuncture, Suite 1, 19A Cavendish Square, London W1M 9AD will send you a register of other lay practitioners, enclose s.a.e. and £1 to cover costs.

Shiatsu and Acupressure

Shiatsu is the Japanese word meaning finger pressure, it's the Japanese form of Acupressure, which basically is acupuncture without the needles. Instead a form of

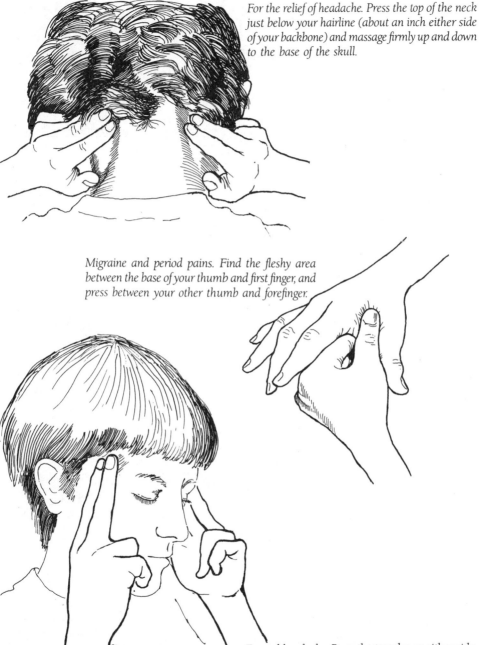

For the relief of headache. Press the top of the neck just below your hairline (about an inch either side of your backbone) and massage firmly up and down to the base of the skull.

Migraine and period pains. Find the fleshy area between the base of your thumb and first finger, and press between your other thumb and forefinger.

Frontal headache. Press the temples on either side between your eyebrow and hair.

Figure 22.

massage using thumbs, hands, elbows and even the knees and feet, is used to rebalance the body's energy.

Treatment lasts an hour to an hour and a half, and may taken place once a week, or less often depending on the condition. You may be treated sitting, kneeling or lying down.

Shiatsu is one of the fastest growing alternative therapies. It's also a simple, easy to learn first-aid technique that can be used in the home for minor ailments such as headaches and period pains, or as a preventive treatment.

Experts say you will feel a sensation midway between pleasure and pain.

Further information:
Shiatsu Society, 19 Langside Park, Kilbarchan, Renfrewshire, PA10, 2EP.

British School of Acupressure Massage, Holistic Healing Centre, 92 Sheering Road, Old Harlow, Essex CM17 0JT. Tel: Harlow 29060.

Acupuncture without Needles by Julian Kenyon, available from the Centre for Study of Alternative Therapies, 51 Bedford Place, Southampton SO1 2DG.

Reflexology (zone therapy/foot massage)

As off-shoot of acupressure, reflexology involves massage and pressure to the soles of the feet, using the hands or a special vibrating device. This is said to stimulate nerve-endings in the feet so provoking a reflex action in other organs or tissues. Practitioners discover problem areas by feeling little chrystal-nodules under the skin on the bottom of the foot. Often problem areas will be uncovered during the massage — for instance if you have bladder problems you will feel tenderness in the arch of your foot. Alternatively you may experience feelings in your bladder when the therapist massages the corresponding area of your foot.

Reflexology is said to help most stress-related disorders. It is extremely relaxing, it can help menstrual problems and those related to the menopause, headache and high blood pressure. It makes a useful adjunct to other types of therapy, or can be used alone.

Further information:
The Bayly School of Reflexology Ltd, Monks Orchard, Whitbourne, Worcester WR6 5RB Tel: 0886 21207.

International Institute of Reflexology, PO Box 34, Harlow, Essex. Tel: Harlow 29060.

Reflexology: A Patient's Guide, Nicola Hall, (Thorsons).

Massage

Massage has been practised in the Far East for thousands of years. It's a simple, pleasurable way to ease aches and pains, aid relaxation, and combat stress. Anyone can do it. You don't have to have any special training.

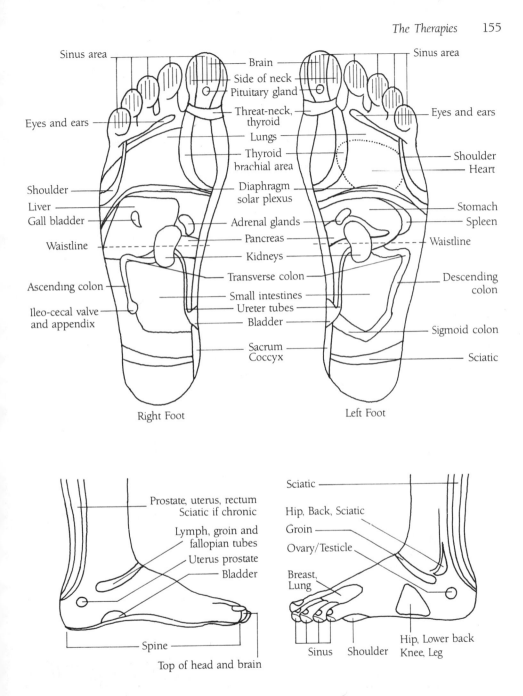

Figure 23: Reflexology zones.

If you go for a massage you can expect the masseur to use a combination of stroking (effleurage), rubbing and kneading.

There's no need to be ill to enjoy a massage. On the other hand, massage can be useful if you are suffering from an illness. Some hospitals include it now as part of their therapy for patients who have had a heart attack.

Finding a suitable masseuse may be a problem for women. Ask around people you know, or if you belong to a gym or sports club ask the organizers if they know of anyone.

Further information:
The Massage Book, by George Downing, (Penguin) is full of useful hints if you want to learn to massage. Here are some of them:

● Apply enough pressure when you massage

● Keep your hands relaxed

● Mould your hands to fit the contours of your partner's body

● Maintain steady speed and pressure

● Explore the underlying structure of your partner's body

● Use your weight rather than muscle power to apply pressure

● Keep in continuous contact with your partner's body throughout the massage

● Massage with your whole body not just your hands

● Don't strain yourself

● Remember your partner is a person and not just a piece of dough!

● Ask your partner what he or she likes best.

Alexander technique

The Alexander principle, named after its founder, a nineteenth century Australian actor F. Matthias Alexander, is a type of therapy designed to change postural habits so as to prevent and treat ill health. Alexander believed that many everyday aches and pains, as well as more serious ill health, arise because of bad habits in the way we hold ourselves, for example hunching over a book, the ironing board, or a factory bench. Treatment consists of a series of lessons to help you learn to hold yourself correctly. A special programme is worked out for you as an individual. Alexander technique is especially helpful for all those vague aches and pains that can make us feel slightly under the weather. It can also help with tiredness, headaches and even childbirth.
Further information:
Society of Teachers of the Alexander Technique, 10 London House, 266 Fulham Road, London SW10 9EL. Tel: 01 351 0828.

Movement therapies

Yoga
Yoga doesn't fall easily into the category of a therapy, as such. Even so it benefits every aspect of the body, mind and spirit, which

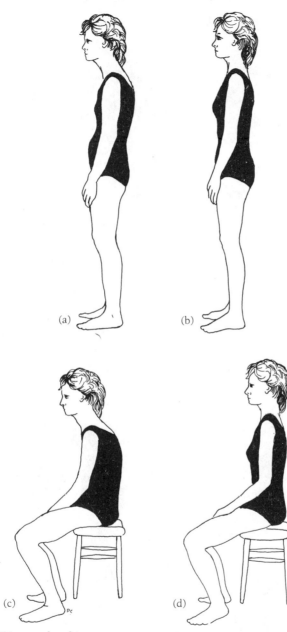

Figure 24: (a) Woman slouching.
(b) Woman standing with body properly aligned.
(c) Sitting collapsed.
(d) Sitting upright.

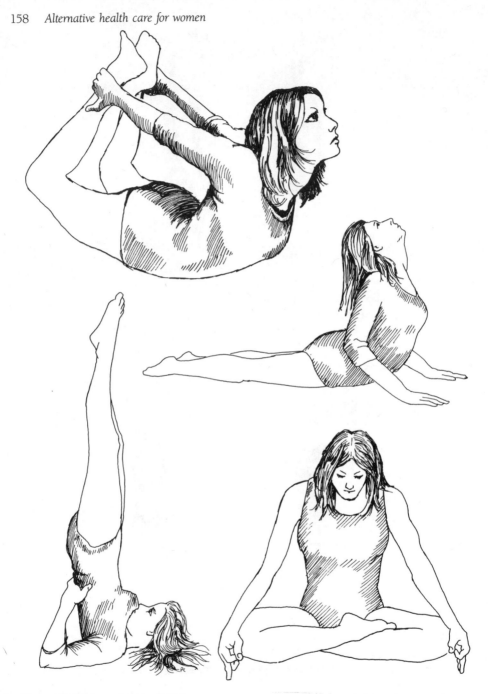

Figure 25: Various yoga postures.

makes it useful as an adjunct to almost any other type of treatment, and also a particularly beneficial form of exercise. The physical practice of yoga consists of asanas (postures) and breathing exercises (pranayama). But yoga is far more than just a system of exercise. The four paths of yoga are:

1. action
2. devotion
3. knowledge and wisdom
4. physical and mental control

Hatha yoga is the type most commonly found in the West. The emphasis in a yoga class will vary according to your teacher, but at least at first the emphasis is on physical and mental control. Once you've learned the techniques you can practice them regularly at home. Yoga is especially useful for combatting and avoiding the effects of stress, which makes it a valuable preventive and treatment for almost any illness.

Further information:
British Wheel of Yoga, 80 Leckhampton Road, Cheltenham, Glos. Tel: 0232 23889.

Iyengar Yoga Institute, 223A Randolph Avenue, London W9 1NL. Tel: 01-624 3080. Many LEAs lay on yoga classes, contact your Adult Education Organizer.

Yoga for Health Foundation, Ickwell Bury, Biggleswade, Bedfordshire SG18 9EF.

T'ai Chi ch'uan
T'ai chi, as it's more usually known, is a form of meditation through movement. You are taught a sequence of gentle flowing actions. In fact if you see T'ai chi in action it's hard to believe that it is in fact a martial art. Above all T'ai chi is slow and gentle. It exercises every part of the body, and leads to increased sense of well being and tranquillity. Because it is non-aggressive it is especially suitable for women and older people or heart patients for whom more active types of movement would be unsuitable.

Further information:
British T'ai Chi Ch'uan Association, 7 Upper Wimpole Street, London W1M 7TD Tel: 01-935 8444.

International T'ai Chi Chu'uan Association, 184/192 Drummond Street, London NW1 Tel: 01-387 5381.

Dance therapy
Dance has been a part of human celebration and ritual for many thousands of years. Dance exercises the body and releases tension. There are far too many forms of dance to go into them all here. Where used as a therapy it is especially useful in helping people to express mental and emotional feelings through their bodies, leading to a sense of release. Dance therapy is used among other places at Charing Cross Hospital with heart patients, and St George's Hospital London with pregnant women. In fact it is especially helpful for anxiety and depression or at any time when you are undergoing major life changes such as during pregnancy, the menopause and so on.

Further information:
The Fitness Jungle, Hetty Einzig and Christopher Connolly, (Century).

The Association for Dance Movement Therapy, 99 South Hill Park, London NW3 Tel: 01-769 0924 or 01-834 4533.

Mind therapies

Psychotherapy

Psychotherapy includes any treatment that uses talking instead of drug treatment. It may be given by a psychiatrist, a medically trained doctor with extra training in psychology, or a psychologist, who has made a study of the mind and its mechanisms.

There are many different approaches to psychotherapy, and it's clearly impossible in a book such as this to go into them all.

Of particular interest to women is feminist psychotherapy which looks at women's problems within a political understanding of what it means to be a woman in our society. For a feminist psychotherapist contact The Women's Therapy Centre, who will put you in touch with someone in your area if possible.

A useful rundown of psychotherapeutic techniques that are commonly used, and can be used as the basis of self-help groups is to be found in *In our Own Hands* by Sheila Ernst and Lucy Goodison, (Women's Press). Because of the many different approaches to psychotherapy it's important to find someone you feel happy with and trust.

It's not easy finding a psychotherapist. You could try asking your doctor, but he will most likely refer you to the local psychiatric service which may well be oversubscribed.

Further information:

MIND, the Association for Mental Health, produces a Psychotherapy List. Send a large s.a.e. marked Psychotherapy list, to the Information Unit, MIND, 22 Harley Street, London W1N 2ED.

The British Association for Counselling, 371 Sheep Street, Rugby, Warwickshire CV1 3AD Tel: Rugby 78328/9 publishes directories on counselling and agencies providing psychotherapy, counselling and support for psychosexual problems.

The Women's Therapy Centre, 6 Manor Gardens, London N7. (Enclose s.a.e.)

Hypnotherapy

Hypnosis is an alternated state of mind. A hypnotist I spoke to described being hypnotized as being akin to the sensation you experience in the moment between sleeping and waking. The hypnotherapist enables this state to be extended, which makes it a useful way to 'unlock' the mind, and therefore it works very well as a form of psychotherapy. You can also be trained to hypnotize yourself (autohypnosis) which can be a useful technique for dealing with stress, pain and so on.

People are often worried that they will be persuaded to do things they wouldn't normally do in everyday life under hypnotism. A fear which is fuelled by the use of hypnotism as a form of popular entertainment. The hypnotist I spoke to assured me this couldn't happen, and that you would automatically snap out of the hypnotic state if you were asked to do something you didn't agree to. However it has to be said that research in this area is contradictory, so be careful who you go to.

Hypnotherapy can be useful in helping you give up smoking, come off tranquillizers, cope with the pain of childbirth, and relieve anxiety, depression, headaches and migraine. A recent report in a medical journal shows it to be effective for some women experiencing repeated miscarriages.

People vary in how suggestible they are, and hypnotherapy doesn't work for everyone. Where it does it can help you deal with problems that are troubling you faster than ordinary psychotherapy by by-passing the barriers we normally put up to defend ourselves against facing troublesome issues.

Many orthodox doctors have now learned hypnotism and your G.P. may be willing to refer you to a reputable non-medical practitioner.

Further information:
British Society for Medical and Dental Hypnosis, 42 Links Road, Ashtead, Surrey, KT21 2HJ (medically trained practitioners).

UK Training College of Hypnotherapy and Counselling, College House, Wrights Lane, London.

Co-counselling
This is a particularly useful therapy for helping you to deal with problems that are bothering you, that perhaps aren't serious enough to warrant professional psychotherapy. Two people take it in turns to counsel each other, taking it in turns to be 'client' and counsellor.

You have to take a special 40 hour induction course to teach you a few simple listening techniques. The basic idea is that by throwing off the restraints normally placed on the expression of feeling by your upbringing, through laughter, tears, trembling, anger, (catharsis) — you can let go of things from your past that are preventing you from living in the present. Its present focus makes it a very positive type of therapy. It's especially suitable for women, since the normal power structure that operates between helper and helped is shared between counsellor and client. However Sheila Ernst & Lucy Goodison mention some reservations in *In Our Own Hands* (Women's Press), 'we feel it gives

too much weight to individual change . . . not enough to confronting external political realities . . . We would also question the emphasis on discharge, which we feel needs to be combined with other things like understanding defences and learning new ways of relating . . . it offers no techniques for the client and counsellor to explore the relationship between them. Emotions can be hived off safely into your hour of discharge.'

Further information:
To find out if there is a local co-counselling group in your area, ask at your local library or CAB. The Women's Therapy Centre, 6 Manor Gardens, London N7, has details of groups including some women-only groups.

Human Potential Research Project, University of Surrey, Guildford GU2 5XH. (Runs induction courses.)

Autogenic training
This is a well-established, effective relaxation method. According to Dr Malcolm Carruthers, who pioneered the technique in this country it involved 'a series of easy mental exercises designed to switch off the stress "fight or flight" system of the body, and switch on the rest, relaxation and recreation system.' The London Autogenic Training Centre says it can help you give up alcohol or smoking, deal with depression, tension, hostility, premenstrual tension and menopausal problems, as well as help you come off tranquillizers, sleeping tablets and so on.

Autogenic training phrases	
My right arm is heavy	Heartbeat calm and regular
My right arm is heavy	Heartbeat calm and regular
My left arm is heavy	Breathing calm and regular
My left arm is heavy	Breathing calm and regular
My right leg is heavy	My centre is warm
My right leg is heavy	My centre is warm
My left leg is heavy	My forehead is cool
My left leg is heavy	My forehead is cool
My arms and legs are heavy and warm	My neck and shoulders are heavy
My arms and legs are heavy and warm	My neck and shoulders are heavy

Further information:
London Autogenic Training Centre, 101 Harley Street, London W1N 1DF.

Biofeedback

Biofeedback is not a therapy as such, but can be used to aid relaxation, yoga, autogenic training. It's a way of monitoring bodily processes such as blood-pressure, heart rate, temperature and muscle tension by means of a gadget, called a biofeedback machine. The machine is usually a little electronic box which gives out a continuous tone or bleep. Two electrodes which measure changes in the body's surface moisture are attached to the palms of your hands. The idea is that when you feel tense or anxious you sweat more — think of the clammy hands you get when you visit the dentist! The machine picks up minute changes in body moisture and the tone emitted rises, when you are calm it falls. In this way you can check when you are really relaxed.

A research trial at St Mary's Hospital, London, has showed that biofeedback can be a useful way of treating pregnant women with a mild degree of hypertension (high blood pressure) (in this study defined as 135/85) rather than the traditional techniques of drugs and complete bed-rest.

You can also use it if you suffer from tension headaches, backache, in fact anything where stress is a component.

Further information:
Local holistic or women's health groups may know of where you can hire or buy equipment in your area.
Audio Ltd, 26 Wendell Road, London W12 9RT give training in the use of their own machines.

Spiritual healing

The ritual of 'laying on of hands' is as old as the human race, and the belief that some people are able to tap into a healing force that can be channelled from the healer to the sick person is not a new one. In fact spiritual healers are one of the few types of alternative therapists who are allowed into NHS hospitals, while a growing number of doctors practise spiritual healing.

Spiritual healing doesn't always involve the 'laying on of hands', it can also be done at a distance.

How does it work?

According to Brian Inglis and Ruth West in *The Alternative Health Guide* (Michael Joseph): 'The hypothesis is that healers have something in their "energy fields" which is capable of interacting with and replenishing the energy fields of patients. How this happens remains a mystery.'

It all sounds too fantastic to be true. Nonetheless throughout the ages there have been anecdotal reports of people being mysteriously healed after contact with a healer. A modern patient, who is also a nurse, provides an example of this, writing in *Nursing Times*, November 20, 1985: 'Twelve months ago Susan Mitchell was told she had between three and five years to live. At 38 Mrs Mitchell was diagnosed a suffering from chronic myeloid leukaemia. . . The only real cure was bone marrow transplantation from a sibling. But Sue Mitchell didn't have one . . . In desperation, she visited the Bristol Cancer Help Centre, which offers holistic treatment, including spiritual healing. Last month, after nine months of regular healing sessions, her doctors at King's told her that her blood count was normal. More rigorous testing revealed a couple of malignant cells, but the blood was virtually clear.' A miracle? Spontaneous remission? Perhaps it doesn't matter what label you stick on it, the point is something worked.

The Confederation of Healing Organizations has recently launched a five year research project in NHS hospitals throughout the country to see whether spiritual healing can help in cases of cataract, rheumatoid arthritis, cancer in children, pain, and a rare joint condition called 'oedime bleu' for which there is no medical treatment. The trial is to be evaluated by independent medical scientists. So perhaps we could soon see some answers to the question of whether it works.

Therapeutic Touch, a modern derivative of laying on of hands, has been subject to trials in America for the treatment of tension headache. The patients who had received TT had an average 70 per cent reduction in pain which carried on over the next four hours, which was greater than a group subjected to placebo.

It seems that like so many healing processes spiritual healing and therapeutic touch could work in some way by reducing stress. One researcher in the USA demonstrated increased haemoglobin levels in patients following therapeutic touch. Patients who have received healing and therapeutic touch report deep feelings of relaxation. But even where such treatments don't affect a cure, and the Federation of Spiritual Healers is the first to say that it doesn't always work, any more than orthodox treatments do, perhaps the feelings of being more relaxed and able to cope count more than anything. The article in the *Nursing Times* has this to say: 'After the session, most of the patients said they felt extremely relaxed and more able to cope with day to day problems. Some felt physical pain relief immediately . . . For some the success of the physical healing was not important. They just wanted somebody to listen to their problems.'

Further information:

The Secretary, National Federation of Spiritual Healing, Old Manor Farm Studio, Church Street, Sunbury on Thames, Middlesex TW16 6RG.

The Centre for Health and Healing, St. James's Church, Piccadilly, London W1.

Incidentally you don't have to belong to a religion or have religious faith to benefit from healing.

Meditation

The image many of us carry around when the word meditation is mentioned is of someone sitting in a flowing robe contemplating a flower. In fact there are many different ways of meditating. Concentrating on an object such as a flower, a vase, a picture is just one. Meditation can incorporate many alternative therapies. Alexander Technique and T'ai Chi, for instance can be ways of reaching a meditative state through the use of the body. It's important to find the way of meditating that suits you as an individual.

Meditation has time and again been shown to have physiological effects. Experienced yogis, can control their blood pressure, heart rate and other bodily processes during meditation. And it's recently been shown that meditation has an effect on the immune system. This could explain its usefulness in preventing and treating illness.

With practice, meditation can help you see the world in a new way, and give you increased energy and enthusiasm. But if you're expecting instant enlightenment, forget it. Holistic doctor Laurence Le Shan says in *How to Meditate* (Turnstone): 'Insight experiences do occur . . . but they are only the beginning . . . After the insight comes the long hard work of following it up: of changing our perceptions, feelings and behaviour to gradually, painfully, bring them into accord with our understanding.'

There are plenty of good books around that can teach you the basics of meditation. Mental meditation, through concentrating on counting your breaths, or a mantra (phrase that you repeat during the meditation), is perhaps the easiest form of meditation to teach yourself. If your 'path of meditation' is through the body, perhaps through dance, yoga, T'ai Chi, or through the practice of a particular skill such as weaving, pottery, singing, you will probably need a teacher. Meditation can also be achieved through your emotions, by 'loosening your feelings.'

As always choose a school of meditation or teacher who appeals to you. Beware of charismatic leaders who claim to be the fount of all wisdom, or possess some special secret knowledge.

Tips for meditating

● Work out how much time you have to give to it. Be realistic.

● Set aside a regular period each day — say 15 to 20 minutes when you know you won't be disturbed.

● Set aside a place for meditating. A warm room where the lighting can be dimmed by drawing the curtains, or switching off the light is suitable.

● Don't meditate immediately after a meal or after drinking coffee, tea or alcohol.

● Allow yourself a few minutes to come to slowly after meditating.

Further information:
How to Meditate, by Laurence Le Shan, (Turnstone Press).

School of Meditation, 158 Holland Park Avenue, London W11 4UH.

Local education authorities often hold meditation classes, look in the prospectuses that come out in the Autumn term, or ring your local adult education organizer.

Table showing illnesses and therapies

This is only a very rough guide. Some of the illnesses will need orthodox treatment as well as alternative. For more details consult the appropriate sections in the book.

KEY: xxx = excellent results
xx = worth a try
x = may be useful as an adjunct to other therapies, orthodox or alternative

Therapies	AIDS	Amenorrhoea	Anaemia	Anxiety	Bartholin cyst	Benign breast disease	Cancer	Cervical erosion	Chlamydia	Cystitis	Depression	Dysmenorrhoea
Acupuncture	xx	xxx		xx		xx	x				xx	xxx
Alexander technique				xx							xx	x
Aromatherapy		xx		x						xx	xx	x
Bach flower remedies				xx			x	x		xx	xx	
Biochemic tissue salts		xx		x							x	x
Biofeedback		xx		xxx								
Chiropractic												
Clinical ecology		xx	xx	xxx		xxx				xxx	x	x
Dance therapy				xxx							xx	x
Herbal medicine	xx	xxx		xxx	xx	xxx	xx	xx	x	xxx	xx	xx
Homoeopathy		xxx		xxx	xx	xx	xx	xx	x	xxx	xx	xx
Hypnotherapy		xx		xxx			xx				xxx	xx
Massage				xxx			xx	xx			xx	x
Meditation/visualization	xx	xx		xxx			xxx	xx		x	xxx	xx
Megavitamin therapy	xx	xx	xxx	xx		xxx	xxx	x		xx	xx	x
Naturopathy	xx	xx	xx	xx	xxx		xxx	xx		xxx	xxx	xx
Osteopathy		xx		x						xx	xx	x
Psychotherapy	xx			xxx			xxx				xxx	x
Reflexology		xx		xx		x		x		xx	xx	x
Shiatsu				xx							x	x
Spiritual healing	xx	xx		xx		x	xxx			xx	xx	
Yoga										xx	xx	xxx

Condition / Therapy	Acupuncture	Alexander technique	Aromatherapy	Bach flower remedies	Biochemic tissue salts	Biofeedback	Chiropractic	Clinical ecology	Dance therapy	Herbal medicine	Homoeopathy	Hypnotherapy	Massage	Meditation/visualization	Megavitamin therapy	Naturopathy	Osteopathy	Psychotherapy	Reflexology	Shiatsu	Spiritual healing	Yoga
Trichomonas										xx	xx			x		x						
Thrush								xx		xxx	xxx		x	x	x	xxx						
Pre-eclampsia						xxx					x	xx		x	x	xx						
Postnatal depression	xx	x	x	x				xx	xx	xx	xx	xx	xx	xx	xxx	xxx	x	xxx	xx		xxx	xxx
PID								xxx		xxx	xxx			xx								
Osteoporosis								xx		xxx					xxx	xxx						
Infertility	xxx							xxx		xxx	xxx	xx		xx	xxx	xxx	xx		x		xxx	
Hot flushes										xxx	xxx			x	xxx	xxx						
Herpes			x							xxx	xxx			xx	xx	xxx			x	xx		
Headache/Migraine	xxx	xxx	xx		xx	xx	xxx	xxx		xxx	xxx	xx	xxx	xx	xx	xxx	xxx	x	xx	xxx	xxx	xxx
Fibroids	xxx						xxx			xxx	xx			xx		xxx		x	xx			
Fatigue	xx	xxx	xx	x				xxx	xxx	x	x	x	x	x	xxx	xxx	xx		xx	xx	xxx	xxx
Endometriosis	xx							xx		xxx	xxx	xx		xxx	xxx	xxx			xx	x		

Index

Other recommended reading . . .
YOUR BODY

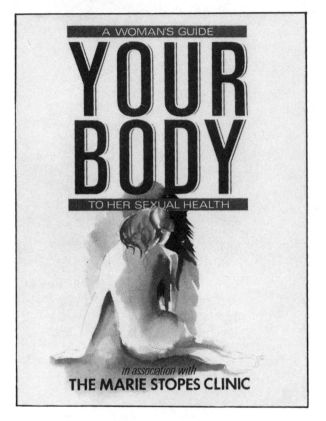

In association with the Marie Stopes Clinic

A Woman's Guide To Her Sexual Health

Designed for the 'new breed of woman' who is aware of herself as an individual, concerned about maintaining her own sexual good health and, above all, no longer content to accept a passive role in any treatment meted out by a male-dominated medical profession. Today's woman is ready to assume responsibility for her *own* physical well-being . . . but to do this she MUST be well-informed and alert to the danger signals her body can provide. This book *gives* such vital information including: self examination; diet and exercise; infertility; sexually transmitted diseases; rape; hysterectomy; personal hygiene.